The Provider Mindset

A Complete Guide to Becoming a Competitive Nurse Anesthesiology Applicant

Leah M. Gordon, DNP, APRN, CRNA

ISBN: 979-8-234-13955-9

DEDICATION

For Grady James,

You give me a reason to do my best every day. I hope this book reminds you that with perseverance, humility, and purpose, anything is possible. Never stop believing in yourself or chasing the dreams that matter most.

Contents

Acknowledgements

Writing a book is never a solitary endeavor. Although my name appears on the cover, this work reflects the encouragement, wisdom, and support of countless people who have shaped both my personal and professional journey. While this is a small book in the world of literature, I want to take a minute to acknowledge those who support me in print.

To my mom and dad, thank you for teaching me the value of hard work, integrity, and striving to do my best every day. Your encouragement, sacrifices, and unshakeable belief in me have shaped the person I am today. Every opportunity I have been given is built upon the foundation you created. Dad, I miss you every day, but I know you are always with me.

To my husband, Beau, thank you for your love, encouragement, and unwavering support. Your patience through the countless hours spent teaching, writing, mentoring, and serving others has made this work possible. Thank you for believing in me, even when my schedule left little room for anything else.

To my sister, Sarah, my forever best friend, thank you for being my first great love. To my brother, Chad; and my sister-in-law, Mandee, thank you for your constant encouragement, your friendship, and for always cheering me on. Having a family that genuinely celebrates one another's successes is a gift I never take for granted.

To my nephews, Landon and Wyatt, you are the world's greatest nephews. You have taught me more than you will ever know, and I am honored to be your aunt.

Aunt Patti, thank you for the career you helped make possible. None of this would have happened without you.

Grandma Gwen and Grandma Behnke, you were two of the brightest lights in my life. I love you, I miss you, and I carry your influence with me every day.

I am deeply grateful to my dear friends and colleagues—Dr. Carol Daniel, Dr. Julie Gauderman, Dr. Elizabeth Gerber, Dr. Lisa Maw, Dr. Amy Heinz, Susan Jarosak, Marlene Kiester, Kati Pownell, & Matthew Lundy. Thank you for your friendship, your honesty, and your willingness to share your wisdom. Each of you has influenced me as an educator, leader, and clinician in ways that extend far beyond the pages of this book.

Thank you to all the individuals who mentored me along the way- Dr. Raj Verma, Dr. Rachel Edgerton, Dr. Todd Walter, Dr. Denise Christie, Dr. Ingrid Anderson, Dr. Danilo Lovinaria, Dr. Roxanne McMurray, and Dr. Paul Kotz. You are my colleagues and friends who inspired me and nurtured me to take risks and keep going when I did not think I could. Thank you for your guidance.

Finally, to the nurse anesthesiology students/ residents of the past, present, and future: thank you. It has been one of the greatest privileges of my career to watch you grow from critical care nurses into anesthesia professionals. You continually challenge me to become a better educator, a better leader, and a better person. Your questions inspire this work, your determination gives it purpose, and your future successes are the reason I continue to teach, write, and advocate for our profession.

I hope this book serves as both a practical guide and a source of encouragement throughout your journey. Becoming a nurse anesthetist/ nurse anesthesiologist requires resilience, humility, discipline, and perseverance—but it is one of the most meaningful and rewarding careers you can pursue. Thank you for allowing me to be a small part of your journey. It has truly been one of the greatest honors of my life.

Introduction

If you've picked up this book, congratulations.

You have made the decision to pursue one of the most challenging—and rewarding—careers in healthcare: nurse anesthesiology.

Whether you are still exploring the profession, preparing your application, or have already been accepted into a program, you are about to begin a journey that will test you academically, professionally, and personally. There will be moments when you question yourself. There will be moments when you wonder if you belong. I hope this book reminds you that those feelings are normal—and that they do not define your potential.

Nurse anesthesiology has a remarkable history. In the earliest days of surgery, anesthesia was not a medical specialty. It was a responsibility entrusted to the surgeon's most capable and dependable nurse. Long before electrocardiograms, pulse oximeters, capnography, or ultrasound, those pioneers relied on careful observation, sound clinical judgment, and unwavering vigilance.

Technology has transformed how we care for patients, but the essence of the profession has not changed. Today, just as then, patients place their lives in our hands. That responsibility is both humbling and extraordinary.

Why I wrote this book

My path to becoming a CRNA was anything but traditional.

As an undergraduate, I graduated with a subpar GPA in Natural Resources. I loved the environment but found little opportunity that would provide sustained employment. A mentor recommended I try working in the hospital while I figured my life out, and it was the best thing that could have happened to me.

Along the way I worked as a Health Unit Coordinator, became an ICU nurse, earned my nursing degrees one step at a time, entered nurse anesthesia school, and eventually discovered that my greatest passion was not only working in healthcare, but also helping others achieve the same dream.

Today, I divide my professional life between clinical practice and education. I continue to care for patients as a practicing CRNA while serving as a program director and educator. Over the years I have reviewed thousands of applications, interviewed hundreds of candidates, celebrated remarkable successes, and walked alongside students through some of the most difficult moments of their careers.

Those experiences have taught me something important.

Admission into nurse anesthesiology school is about far more than grades, certifications, or checking boxes. The strongest applicants are rarely perfect. They are resilient. They are reflective. They seek feedback, learn from setbacks, and continue moving forward even when the path becomes difficult.

That is the person admissions committees are looking for.

A Little About Me

I also believe it's important that you know something about the person writing this book. I grew up in Forest Lake, Minnesota, and have spent my entire professional career in healthcare, working in and around the Twin Cities Metro area.

I also live with a physical disability—foot drop caused by peroneal nerve damage. Although it has never defined me, it has shaped how I view perseverance, adaptability, and the importance of seeing the whole person rather than a single characteristic. I am the first one to want the disadvantaged to succeed, and I am so grateful to lead a school where I can help make that a reality.

My personal and professional life have also been shaped by the diverse communities I have been privileged to serve.

Working in Minneapolis during times of profound social change has reinforced the importance of humility, listening, cultural awareness, and recognizing that every patient and every student brings a unique story and perspective. Those experiences continue to influence how I practice, how I teach, and how I lead.

I did not arrive here alone.

Like many people, I had mentors who recognized something in me before I recognized it in myself. My Auntie Patti first encouraged me to consider nursing and introduced me to the opportunity that became the beginning of my healthcare career. My parents supported me while I pursued a second degree.

As a Health Unit Coordinator who worked throughout nursing school, I learned medicine from the ground up—working alongside nurses, physicians, respiratory therapists, and countless others who generously shared their knowledge. Every stage of my career has been shaped by people willing to invest in someone who was still learning.

I hope this book can be one small way of doing the same for you. Just reading it is one small step towards your goal.

Why Listen to Me?

There are countless resources available for aspiring CRNAs. Some are excellent. Others promise shortcuts, formulas, or "secrets" to getting accepted into school.

This book is different.

Everything you will read comes from the perspective of someone who has spent years teaching, interviewing applicants, serving on admissions committees, mentoring students, and leading a highly successful accredited nurse anesthesiology program while continuing to practice clinically. I think anyone who works in education has taken the pay cut to prove that they care more about the profession, the students, and the process of education over their own pocketbook.

I don't believe there is a secret formula for getting accepted, and if you just pay enough money, you will get the recipe.

I do believe there is tremendous value in understanding what admissions committees are truly looking for, how successful applicants distinguish themselves, and how to avoid the common mistakes that keep otherwise qualified candidates from reaching their goals.

My hope is that this book helps you spend less time (and money) trying to determine what schools want and more time becoming the provider you aspire to be.

That being said... If there is one lesson I hope you remember, it is this:

Hard things almost always take longer than you think they will.

Your application may take longer to build than you expected. It may take longer than you want to get accepted into a program. There are MANY qualified candidates and not enough spots to educate them all. Give yourself some grace. You are enough as you are. There will be days when you wonder whether you belong. Keep going.

The profession needs knowledgeable clinicians. It needs compassionate leaders. It needs people who are willing to do difficult things well.

Perhaps most importantly, it needs people who understand that excellence is not achieved overnight—it is built one patient, one lesson, one challenge, and one day at a time.

Welcome to the journey.

Terminology

Throughout this book, I use the terms nurse anesthetist and nurse anesthesiologist interchangeably when referring to Certified Registered Nurse Anesthetists (CRNAs). Likewise, I use the terms student registered nurse anesthetist (SRNA) and resident registered nurse anesthetist (RRNA) interchangeably when referring to individuals enrolled in nurse anesthesiology educational programs.

My choice of terminology is not intended to advocate for one title over another or to suggest a particular position in ongoing professional discussions. Rather, it reflects the reality that multiple terms are currently used throughout our profession, often influenced by state laws, institutional policies, educational programs, historical context, and personal preference.

The decision to use one term instead of another is rarely simple. It is shaped by legal, regulatory, professional, and cultural considerations that continue to evolve. My goal is not to wade into those debates, but to communicate clearly with readers from a variety of backgrounds who may be more familiar with one term than another.

Throughout this book, I generally use the term **nurse anesthesiology** rather than **nurse anesthesia**. This is an intentional choice.

To me, *anesthesiology* refers to the scientific discipline and practice of providing anesthesia care—a body of knowledge that is advanced through the contributions of CRNAs, physicians, researchers, educators, and countless others. I believe the science of anesthesiology belongs to all who have dedicated their careers to its advancement.

I recognize that both terms are widely accepted and commonly used throughout the profession, and my choice of terminology should not be interpreted as criticism of those who prefer one term over the other. It simply reflects the language that I feel most accurately describes the profession and the science that unite us.

Regardless of the terminology used, my respect for our profession and the individuals who practice it remains the same. I encourage readers to focus not on the title, but on the professionalism, competence, compassion, and commitment to patient care that define nurse anesthesia providers and the students preparing to join this remarkable profession.

Part I: Starting the Journey to your Nurse Anesthesiology Degree

The nurse anesthesiology profession is unique in many ways, beginning with the path required to enter it. It is difficult to identify another profession in which individuals must first complete post-secondary education, then enter the workforce and progress into one of the most complex and high-stakes roles within an organization—critical care nursing—only to step away and return to full-time graduate education. Even in programs that offer "direct admission," there remain clear expectations and milestones that must be met before matriculation. There is no shortcut to anesthesia school—only a path defined by sustained effort, discipline, and commitment to the goal.

As I write this, I find myself revisiting the work of nurse scholars and educators who came before me. The breadth of their contributions is vast, but I am continually drawn back to the history of nursing—the layers of progress, challenge, advocacy, and at times, inequity—that have shaped our profession. These themes will surface throughout this text, because they provide essential context for understanding who you are as a registered nurse today, and who you are becoming as a future anesthesia provider.

Nurses are, in many ways, experts in quiet excellence. We are so skilled at what we do that our work often goes unseen. There is even nursing theory built around this concept of invisibility. Yet here you are, preparing to do something that may feel fundamentally uncomfortable: to step forward, to be seen, and to present yourself as a competitive applicant to a nurse anesthesiology program.

So how do we reconcile that tension?

I would argue that the answer lies in balance. This journey requires both introspection and intentional growth. You must look inward—developing a deep understanding of your motivations, strengths, and areas for growth—while also looking outward, educating yourself about the profession of nursing and the rich, complex history of anesthesiology. It is through this dual awareness that you begin to prepare—not just for admission into a program, but for the responsibility and identity of becoming a nurse anesthesiologist.

Much of this history remains hidden. Medical advances are, by their nature, advances in medicine, and physicians have understandably been central figures in documenting and promoting many of those discoveries. However, the history of nursing tells a different story—one that is deeply intertwined with the evolving role of women in society.

As a profession composed primarily of women for most of its history, nursing has often advanced alongside broader cultural shifts rather than through scientific breakthroughs alone. The struggle for professional recognition, educational advancement, leadership opportunities, and autonomy has reflected society's changing views of women in the workforce. Considering the history of the world, the majority of these changes have happened in the last 50 years. These are important chapters in healthcare history, yet they are often overlooked and not appreciated

It took me many years working in healthcare to realize that most other healthcare professionals are never asked to study the history of nursing. They do not learn that nurses have been providing anesthesia care since the specialty was first developed. They are rarely taught about the decades of advocacy, legislative battles, educational reform, and professional perseverance that have allowed nurse anesthesiology to become the respected profession it is today.

Historically, organized medicine has largely been physician-led and, for much of its existence, male-led. While that leadership has contributed enormously to the advancement of healthcare, it has also, at times, unintentionally minimized the contributions of other professions. I believe healthcare is strongest when every profession's history, expertise, and perspective are recognized and valued. I hope to see continued progress toward that vision during my lifetime.

One of the most meaningful ways we can contribute to the future of nurse anesthesiology is by ensuring that we continue to attract, educate, and graduate exceptional students. Every highly qualified nurse anesthesiologist who enters the profession strengthens not only patient care but also the legacy of those who fought to establish and protect our profession.

What Is Motivating You to Do This?

It was a typical day in procedural care. I was working with a traditional team: a proceduralist, a registered nurse, and me—the nurse anesthetist. My role was to safely monitor and sedate patients undergoing colonoscopies and upper endoscopies in a fast-paced center, where we completed a case every 30 minutes. We were midway through our fifth case of the morning, moving at a steady pace, completing procedures on time.

In the middle of a case, the proceduralist leaned over to the circulating procedure room nurse and casually asked, "Have you ever thought about going to anesthesia school? Why don't you do this?"

There were three of us in the room, all actively caring for a patient who was asleep. There is no doubt that I play a pivotal role in keeping our room moving at a steady pace, based on how quickly I can put the patient to sleep and help them emerge from anesthesia.

From the outside, I knew what it looked like. I make induction and emergence appear smooth, controlled—even easy. I smiled and offered a light response about how wonderful it is to be a CRNA, not quite addressing the deeper implication behind the question—that this was a simple, carefree career one might just decide to pursue.

But later, I couldn't stop thinking about it.

Why do people believe that becoming a CRNA is a casual decision—something you wake up one day and simply choose? How is it possible that even those we work alongside don't fully understand the depth of our profession?

The reality is, our history is rich, complex, and hard-earned. Our role has been shaped through decades of advocacy, resilience, and clinical excellence. And even now, there is constant pressure—external forces that challenge our scope, our value, and our place in healthcare.

This is not a profession you stumble into.

Not everyone can do this. And just as importantly, not everyone should. The pathway is intentionally rigorous, layered with academic, clinical, and professional expectations designed to ensure that those who enter this field are prepared to carry its weight.

So when you ask yourself, *what is motivating you to do this?*—the answer must go deeper than curiosity or convenience.

Because this journey will ask more of you than you may realize.

Reflection Questions

1. What first sparked your interest in nurse anesthesiology, and what about it continues to hold your attention?

2. What parts of your current nursing role feel most meaningful or energizing to you, and how might those connect to anesthesia practice?
3. As you think about your future, what kind of nurse—and person—are you hoping to become?

The Decisional balance: Money, barriers, fears, family, partners, friends

As you begin to build your why, you will find yourself asking about these issues as we go. I will go into this later in the book. I bring it up here though as a touchpoint, because of how important it is. Each of these topics will take some personal exploration on your part. I will touch on them and talk about things I have observed over my 15 years as a CRNA. Ultimately, these are things that you will weigh, and they will continue to come up while you are in school and beyond.

How do you learn?

As you begin to understand *why* you want to return to school, the next logical question becomes: Where do you want to go?

One of the most important—and often overlooked—considerations is how you learn best.

One of the questions I am asked most often is whether our program is "front-loaded." Rather than answering immediately, I usually respond with a question of my own:

What does front-loaded mean to you?

The reality is that the term means different things to different people. Does it mean one semester of classroom learning before entering clinical? Two semesters? An entire year? In today's world of 36-month nurse anesthesiology programs, there is no universally accepted definition, yet applicants often place tremendous importance on the label.

Even if we define a front-loaded curriculum as one in which most of the foundational science and didactic coursework occurs early in the program, the truth is that no nurse anesthesiology program is truly front-loaded.

Why?

Because learning never stops.

The expectation to study, integrate new knowledge, and develop clinical judgment continues throughout every semester of your education. As your clinical responsibility increases, so does the complexity of the knowledge you must master. Every lecture, every clinical experience, and every patient encounter builds upon the one before it. Ultimately, all of that learning culminates in the National Certification Examination (NCE), which every future CRNA must successfully pass.

That is the reality of nurse anesthesiology education.

This journey is not a sprint—it is a 36-month marathon.

The students who are most successful are rarely those who can study the hardest for a few weeks. They are the ones who establish consistent habits, maintain discipline, and continue learning even when life becomes busy or stressful. Your ability to sustain that effort over three years is far more important than whether a program is labeled "front-loaded."

As you compare programs, I encourage you to look beyond the terminology and carefully review each curriculum. Pay particular attention to the first semester. If you notice a very heavy academic load—perhaps 16 or more graduate credits—ask questions. How is the curriculum structured? What academic support is available? How do students typically perform during that first semester? What are the program's attrition and graduation rates?

Some programs intentionally begin with an especially rigorous first semester to establish a strong scientific foundation before students enter clinical practice. Others spread the coursework more evenly across the curriculum. Neither approach is inherently better, but each requires a different learning style and level of preparation.

The goal is not to find the "easiest" curriculum. The goal is to find the program whose structure best matches the way you learn, your support system, and the environment in which you are most likely to thrive.

Critical Care Nurse Learning Styles Assessment

As part of this work to prepare you for anesthesia school, I want to sprinkle self-assessments and self-reflection questions throughout where appropriate. For as much as I want to share my insights with you about nurse anesthesiology education, I also want you to get to know yourself. This first assessment is an opportunity for you to determine the learning style that most represents you.

Instructions: Read each question and circle the answer that most represents how you generally behave in your clinical practice.

1. When I'm learning to use a new piece of ICU equipment (e.g., ventilator, infusion pump), I prefer to:

a) Read the manual, diagrams, or quick reference guide

b) Listen to a colleague or educator explain it

c) Get hands-on and try it out while someone supervises

2. When I receive a complex handoff at shift change, I:

a) Rely on the written flowsheet and visual trends in the EMR

b) Focus on the verbal report and discussion

c) Go to the bedside and check lines, pumps, and monitors myself

3. When orienting to a new procedure (e.g., arterial line insertion, ECMO circuit care), I like to:

a) Watch a video, look at diagrams, or read the step-by-step guide

b) Have someone explain it to me step by step

c) Practice it directly (with supervision if needed)

4. If I'm precepting a new nurse in the ICU, I usually:

a) Write or draw instructions/checklists for them

b) Talk them through the process out loud

c) Demonstrate the skill, then have them try it

5. When a patient is decompensating, I tend to:

a) Scan the monitor, labs, and EHR for visual cues

b) Listen carefully to alarms, staff input, and physician instructions

c) Put hands on the patient, troubleshoot lines/equipment, and act quickly

6. When attending an educational in-service, I remember best if:

a) There are charts, slides, and visual aids

b) The instructor explains clearly and I can ask questions

c) I get to practice with equipment or do a simulation

7. When troubleshooting a ventilator alarm, I first:

a) Look at the waveforms and settings on the screen

b) Ask respiratory therapy or listen to others explain what's happening

c) Assess the patient and tubing hands-on to find the problem

8. If a physician gives new orders in a rapid sequence, I:

a) Prefer to see them written or entered in the chart

b) Like to hear them repeated clearly out loud

c) Start setting up and carrying out the interventions

9. When preparing for certification exams (e.g., CCRN), I:

a) Make study guides, mind maps, and review charts/graphics

b) Use audio lectures, group discussions, or explain concepts aloud

c) Do practice questions, case studies, and simulations

10. If I'm remembering a critical care case, I most often recall:

a) The monitor readings, labs, and what I saw visually

b) The words exchanged in report or physician instructions

c) What I physically did — turning, suctioning, adjusting drips

Scoring:

Count how many A's (Visual), B's (Auditory), and C's (Kinesthetic) you selected. The style with the highest total is your primary learning preference. Many ICU nurses have a blend of two or more styles.

Interpretation for Critical Care Nursing

Visual learners:

Excel with algorithms, flowcharts, ventilator waveforms, ECG strips, and checklists. These learners often thrive in nurse anesthesia programs that emphasize structured didactic content, clear visual aids, organized slide decks, and strong use of simulation visuals or recorded lectures. Programs with well-developed online or hybrid platforms—where material can be reviewed repeatedly—may be especially appealing.

Auditory learners:

Benefit from SBAR handoff, podcasts, discussion-based learning, and teaching peers. These learners may be drawn to programs that prioritize in-person lectures, case discussions, oral boards-style teaching, and collaborative learning environments. Programs with strong faculty engagement, open dialogue, and opportunities to verbalize clinical reasoning can enhance their success.

Kinesthetic learners:

Thrive in simulation labs, hands-on skills (line insertions, codes), and bedside practice. These learners often do best in programs with early and frequent clinical exposure, high-fidelity simulation, and robust skills lab experiences. Programs that emphasize experiential learning, procedural repetition, and immersive clinical practice will align well with their strengths.

Reflection Questions:

1. Think about a time in the ICU when something finally "clicked" for you.
   What helped you understand it—seeing it, hearing it explained, or doing it yourself?
2. When you are under pressure (a code, a rapid change in patient status), how do you learn best in that moment?
   Do you rely on mental checklists and visuals, talking it through, or hands-on action?
3. How do you typically prepare for high-stakes exams or certifications?
   Do you gravitate toward videos and diagrams, recorded lectures and discussion, or practice questions and simulation?
4. When choosing a nurse anesthesia program, what environment will challenge you—but also support how you naturally learn? Are you looking for structure and visual organization, discussion and mentorship, or immersive, hands-on experience?

Part II: The school search

History of Nurse Anesthesiology Education

I have always enjoyed learning about the history of nursing and nurse anesthesiology because understanding where we came from helps us better appreciate where we are today. Our profession did not simply appear overnight in response to a need for anesthesia personnel. It was built over generations by nurses who believed that patients deserved safe, compassionate, and skilled anesthesia care.

Nursing has historically fought to be recognized as an essential profession rather than simply a supporting role. That struggle was reflected in anesthesia as well. During the American Civil War, nurses began administering anesthesia on the battlefield under the direction of surgeons. In the decades that followed, nurse anesthetists became indispensable members of surgical teams, developing extraordinary expertise through repetition, observation, and an unwavering commitment to patient safety.

Many of the innovations that define modern anesthesia can be traced directly to nurse anesthetists. One remarkable example is Betty E. Lank, CRNA (1904–2011), a pioneer of pediatric nurse anesthesiology. During her 34-year career at Boston Children's Hospital, she helped transform the care of infants and children at a time when pediatric anesthesia was still in its infancy. She was the first to use cyclopropane anesthesia in infants, designed child-sized anesthesia masks and ventilation bags, helped establish one of the nation's first pediatric post-anesthesia recovery units, and educated generations of clinicians. Her work demonstrated that nurse anesthetists were not simply delivering anesthesia—they were advancing the science and practice of anesthesia itself.

One of the most influential centers in the development of nurse anesthesiology education was the Mayo Clinic. What began as an apprenticeship model gradually evolved into a structured educational system grounded in science, clinical experience, and accountability. Visionary physicians, including Dr. John Lundy, recognized the value of highly trained nurse anesthetists and supported the development of formal educational standards. At the same time, experienced nurse anesthetists became educators and mentors, passing their knowledge to the next generation while helping define the profession itself.

No discussion of our history would be complete without recognizing Alice Magaw (1860-1928), often referred to as the "Mother of Anesthesia." Working at the Mayo Clinic in the late nineteenth and early twentieth centuries, she safely administered thousands of anesthetics while meticulously documenting her outcomes. At a time when anesthesia was still evolving, her published results demonstrated that carefully trained nurse anesthetists could provide exceptionally safe, consistent care. Her emphasis on vigilance, preparation, and continuous patient observation remains foundational to anesthesia practice today.

The growth of nurse anesthesiology also depended on visionary educators who recognized that the future of the profession required formal training rather than apprenticeship alone. In 1909 Agnes McGee established one of the nation's earliest schools of nurse anesthesia at St. Vincent's Hospital in Portland Oregan, helping create a structured educational pathway for future nurse anesthetists. Her commitment to rigorous clinical preparation demonstrated that excellence in anesthesia could be intentionally taught, setting a standard that influenced nurse anesthesia education for generations.

As educational programs expanded across the country, Helen Lamb, CRNA (1899-1979), helped strengthen the profession through scholarship and communication.

As the first editor of the *AANA Journal*, Lamb promoted the sharing of clinical knowledge, research, and educational best practices at a time when few opportunities existed for nurse anesthetists to learn from one another beyond their own hospitals. McGee, Lamb, and countless other early nurse anesthetists helped transform nurse anesthesiology from a collection of talented individual practitioners into a profession grounded in education, collaboration, and lifelong learning.

Another giant in our profession was Agatha Hodgins (1877-1945), one of the founders of the American Association of Nurse Anesthesiology (AANA). Hodgins recognized that the future of nurse anesthetists would depend not only on excellent patient care but also on professional organization, education, and advocacy. She understood that the language used in legislation and public policy could either strengthen or diminish the profession. Throughout her career, she advocated for terminology that accurately reflected the education, judgment, and responsibility of nurse anesthetists. Her work reminds us that words matter. The language used to describe our profession influences how others perceive us, how laws are written, and ultimately how patients gain access to care.

Much of this history remains hidden. Medical advances are, by their nature, advances in medicine, and physicians have understandably been central figures in documenting and promoting many of those discoveries.

However, the history of nursing tells a different story—one that is deeply intertwined with the evolving role of women in society.

As a profession composed primarily of women for most of its history, nursing has often advanced alongside broader cultural shifts rather than through scientific breakthroughs alone. The struggle for professional recognition, educational advancement, leadership opportunities, and autonomy has reflected society's changing views of women in the workforce. These are important chapters in healthcare history, yet they are often overlooked.

It took me many years working in healthcare to realize that most other healthcare professionals are never asked to study the history of nursing. They do not learn that nurses have been providing anesthesia care since the specialty was first developed. They are rarely taught about the decades of advocacy, legislative battles, educational reform, and professional perseverance that have allowed nurse anesthesiology to become the respected profession it is today.

Historically, organized medicine has largely been physician-led and, for much of its existence, male-led. While that leadership has contributed enormously to the advancement of healthcare, it has also, at times, unintentionally minimized the contributions of other professions.

I believe healthcare is strongest when every profession's history, expertise, and perspective are recognized and valued. I hope to see continued progress toward that vision during my lifetime.

One of the most meaningful ways we can contribute to the future of nurse anesthesiology is by ensuring that we continue to attract, educate, and graduate exceptional students. Every highly qualified nurse anesthesiologist who enters the profession strengthens not only patient care but also the legacy of those who fought to establish and protect our profession.

As you begin your own journey into nurse anesthesiology, remember that you are joining a profession built by individuals who continually challenged expectations. They earned trust through preparation, competence, humility, and outstanding patient care. Those same qualities remain the foundation of our profession today, and they are the qualities you should strive to develop throughout your own education and career.

I often remind my students that the provider mindset did not begin with us. It was passed from one generation of nurse anesthetists to the next through teaching, mentorship, and a relentless commitment to excellence. Now, it is your turn to carry that legacy forward.

AANA DATA

According to the Council on Accreditation of Nurse Anesthesia Educational Programs (COA), as of 2026 there are 155 accredited nurse anesthesiology educational programs in the United States and Puerto Rico. That number has been slowly increasing over the years.

DNP, DNAP, and Choosing the Right Program

One of the questions I hear most often from prospective students is:

"Should I apply to a DNP program or a DNAP program?"

It's a fair question. You're investing three years of your life, taking on a significant financial commitment, and preparing for a profession you'll likely practice for decades. Naturally, you want to make the best decision possible.

The good news is this:

The letters behind the degree are probably much less important than you think.

I have reviewed thousands of applications, interviewed hundreds of candidates, and worked alongside graduates from nurse anesthesiology programs across the country. Never have I looked at an outstanding clinician and thought, "They're an excellent CRNA because they earned a DNP instead of a DNAP."

Outstanding providers graduate from both.

That doesn't mean the degree itself is unimportant. It simply means that when you're comparing programs, there are much more meaningful factors to consider. We'll discuss those later in this chapter, but first it helps to understand why nurse anesthesiology transitioned to the doctoral level.

Why Did Nurse Anesthesiology Move to the Doctoral Degree?

Practice-focused doctoral education in nursing has been evolving for decades. The first practice doctorate in nursing, the Doctor of Nursing (ND), was introduced at Case Western Reserve University in 1979. In 2004, the American Association of Colleges of Nursing (AACN) endorsed the Doctor of Nursing Practice (DNP) as the terminal practice degree for advanced nursing practice.

This transition was never about adding another credential to the end of a name.

Healthcare itself was changing.

Patients were living longer with increasingly complex medical conditions. Technology was advancing rapidly. Healthcare systems were becoming more sophisticated, and the expectation for healthcare providers expanded well beyond direct patient care.

Advanced practice nurses were increasingly expected to lead quality improvement initiatives, evaluate scientific evidence, improve patient safety, educate others, and influence healthcare policy.

Nurse anesthesiology evolved alongside those changes.

Today's CRNAs are expected to be expert clinicians, critical thinkers, leaders, educators, scholars, and advocates for their patients and profession. Modern nurse anesthesiology education reflects those expectations.

Personally, I hope the day comes when we no longer feel compelled to classify providers as "advanced practice" or the mediocre term "mid-level." Those labels do little to describe the responsibility we assume every day. Regardless of title, every patient deserves a clinician who is knowledgeable, prepared, humble, and committed to lifelong learning. That is the standard we should all strive to meet.

Whether you ultimately earn a DNP or a DNAP, your degree is only the beginning. Your competence, professionalism, judgment, and commitment to continual growth are what will define you as a nurse anesthesiologist—not the letters embroidered on your white coat.

What's the Difference Between a DNP and a DNAP?

Although the names are different, both degrees prepare graduates to enter nurse anesthesiology practice at the doctoral level.

The Doctor of Nursing Practice (DNP) is a nursing doctorate designed for all advanced practice registered nurses, including nurse practitioners, nurse midwives, clinical nurse specialists, and CRNAs.

The DNP curriculum emphasizes advanced clinical practice, leadership, evidence-based practice, healthcare policy, quality improvement, and systems thinking across nursing specialties.

The Doctor of Nurse Anesthesia Practice (DNAP) is designed specifically for nurse anesthesiology. While it covers many of the same leadership and scholarly competencies as the DNP, its coursework and scholarly work are centered entirely on anesthesia practice, patient safety, perioperative care, and anesthesia-specific systems leadership.

Think of it this way:

The DNP is a broad advanced practice nursing doctorate.

The DNAP is a specialty doctorate built specifically around nurse anesthesiology.

Neither degree is "better." They're simply different educational models. Both the DNP and the DNAP are accredited by the COA, and both degrees are held to identical educational standards.

Who Decides Which Degree a School Awards?

Many applicants assume that every nurse anesthesiology program must award the same doctoral degree.

That isn't true.

The COA requires that all entry-level nurse anesthesiology programs award a doctoral degree. However, the COA does not require programs to award either a DNP or a DNAP.

That decision belongs to each individual university.

Some universities already educate multiple types of advanced practice nurses and therefore award the DNP to all of their doctoral nursing students. Other institutions have developed an anesthesia-specific doctorate and award the DNAP.

In reality, this decision often reflects the structure and philosophy of the university rather than a difference in educational quality.

What should You Really be Comparing?

If I could give every applicant one piece of advice, it would be this:

Don't choose a school because of the degree title. Instead, compare the things that will actually influence your education. Of course, I don't expect you to know what that is off the top of your head. Sure, it matters where the clinical sites are, and if the Program Director is nice or not (I am sure they are), but there are many things that you should consider.

Ask questions like:

- How many clinical cases will I complete?
- How many facilities will I rotate through?

- Does this program offer simulation experiences?
- What is the faculty-to-student relationship like?
- How does the school support student wellness?
- How are struggling students supported?
- What is the culture of the program?
- Where do graduates find employment?
- Does this program fit my learning style and my career goals?

Those answers will tell you far more about the quality of your future education than whether your diploma says DNP or DNAP

Where Should You Get Your Information?

Today, there is no shortage of websites claiming to compare nurse anesthesiology programs. As a Program Director, companies frequently contact me asking me to review their websites or verify that the information they're publishing about programs is accurate. While I appreciate what they're trying to accomplish, I simply don't have the time to fact-check dozens of third-party websites, especially when program requirements change regularly.

My advice is simple:

Go directly to the source.

Start with the COA website (www.coacrna.org). Every accredited nurse anesthesiology program is required to maintain current information there. Once you've identified programs that interest you, visit each program's official website for the most current admission requirements, curriculum, clinical experiences, tuition, board pass rates, and program outcomes.

Third-party websites can be helpful for general guidance, but they should never be your final authority.

My Final Thoughts On How To Choose

Choosing a nurse anesthesiology program is one of the most important professional decisions you will ever make. I remember when I got into a program, someone told me to take the first offer I got, because you may not get another one. Not bad advice, but I have wondered what I missed out on over the years, since I didn't really look that closely at the program I went to. I honestly think I was lucky, because we didn't have access to information like today's students do. Do your homework. You won't ever feel you wasted your time.

Choose a program that will challenge you, support you, develop your clinical judgment, prepare you to pass boards, and ultimately help you become the safest, most competent nurse anesthesiologist you can be.

The degree matters, but the education behind it matters even more.

What Do Schools Look For?

This is the million-dollar question—and probably the one I am asked more than any other.

After reviewing thousands of applications, interviewing hundreds of candidates, and serving as a nurse anesthesiology program director, I have learned that every applicant brings a unique story. No two applications are exactly alike.

Yet when I strip everything else away, I find myself coming back to two fundamental qualities:

Aptitude and Attitude.

Aptitude

Can you do the work?

Nurse anesthesiology is academically demanding. Programs need evidence that you can master advanced physiology, pharmacology, chemistry, physics, pathophysiology, and complex clinical decision-making.

We evaluate your academic record, ICU experience, certifications, professional development, and your ability to think critically under pressure. Strong grades certainly help, but they are only one piece of the puzzle. We are trying to determine whether you have demonstrated the ability to learn difficult material and apply it safely to patient care.

The truth is, that is not always easy to assess.

Attitude

Will you be someone people want to teach? This is the part many applicants underestimate.

The strongest students are not always the ones with the highest GPA or the longest ICU résumé. They are the ones who are humble enough to accept feedback, resilient enough to recover from mistakes, curious enough to keep asking questions, and professional enough to place the needs of their patients and team ahead of their own ego.

Programs invest thousands of hours in every student they admit. Faculty members, clinical coordinators, and preceptors want to spend those hours teaching someone who is dependable, coachable, hardworking, respectful, and kind.

Knowledge can be taught.

Character is much more difficult to develop.

Ultimately, every admissions committee is trying to answer one question:

"If we invest the next three years in this individual, will they become the kind of CRNA we would trust to care for our own family?"

Every part of your application helps answer that question. Your transcript. Your résumé. Your essay. Your letters of recommendation. Your interview. Even the professionalism you demonstrate in your emails and interactions with admissions staff contributes to the overall picture.

Your goal is not simply to convince a program that you are intelligent enough to succeed.

Your goal is to demonstrate that you possess both the aptitude to thrive academically and the attitude to become an exceptional nurse anesthesiologist.

Artificial Intelligence and the Application Process

I would be remiss if I did not mention the growing role of artificial intelligence in higher education, including the admissions process. Universities are increasingly exploring ways to use technology to assist with administrative tasks such as reviewing applications, identifying trends, and improving efficiency.

Some companies are developing AI-assisted tools that aim to help admissions committees evaluate applicants in a more structured and consistent manner.

These technologies are still in their early stages, and their adoption varies considerably from one institution to another. They are not inexpensive, and many schools may choose not to implement them for years, if ever. Even where AI is used, admissions decisions continue to rely on human judgment, particularly in highly competitive healthcare programs where qualities such as professionalism, communication, and leadership are difficult to measure with technology alone.

My goal is not to make you worry about whether a particular school uses AI. Rather, I want you to recognize that the admissions landscape is evolving. The strongest applications have always been those that are authentic, thoughtful, and supported by real accomplishments. Whether your application is first reviewed by a person, assisted by technology, or some combination of the two, genuine experiences, clear writing, and professional integrity will continue to matter.

If there is one message I hope you take from this chapter, it is this:

Programs are not simply selecting students. They are selecting future colleagues.

Become the kind of person others want beside them in the operating room, and you will have already taken one of the most important steps toward becoming a successful CRNA.

REVIEW QUESTIONS:

1. How might factors such as finances, family, and personal fears influence your decision to pursue anesthesia school, and how do you plan to navigate them?
2. After reviewing the differences between degree options (DNP, DNAP, etc.), how would you approach evaluating programs to find the best fit for your goals?
3. Imagine you are serving on an admissions committee. What evidence in your current application demonstrates your **aptitude**? What evidence demonstrates your **attitude**? Which areas could you strengthen before you apply?
4. Take a few moments to write down questions that you think would be good general questions to ask admissions committee members. Then, take the time to ensure you cannot find those answers on a school's website before you ask.

Part III: The Application Process

Preparing your Resume

Your resume is one of the most important components of your graduate school application. Long before you have the opportunity to interview, it introduces the admissions committee to your education, experience, leadership, certifications, and professional accomplishments. In many ways, it tells the story of how your career has prepared you for advanced practice.

Most applicants already have a resume, and that is an excellent place to start. Before submitting your application, take the time to refine it so that admissions committees can quickly identify the information that matters most. The easier you make it for reviewers to understand your qualifications, the stronger your application will be.

Some applicants also have a curriculum vitae (CV), but for the majority of nurses applying to nurse anesthesiology school, a well-organized resume is all that is needed.

If you get nothing from this book, start working on your resume now. Treat it like a living document that you update on a schedule. Take a look at it once every few months and make sure it is completely current. You will never regret keeping track of your professional life in an organized fashion, no matter where life takes you.

Resume vs. CV

One of the first decisions applicants face is whether to submit a resume or a curriculum vitae (CV).

Resume

A resume is a concise, targeted summary of your qualifications. It is designed for a specific purpose—in this case, admission to a nurse anesthesiology program. Most resumes are one to two pages in length and emphasize the experiences most relevant to the position or program.

Curriculum Vitae (CV)

A curriculum vitae (CV) is a comprehensive record of your professional career. It typically includes your education, employment history, presentations, publications, research, committee work, awards, teaching experience, volunteer activities, professional memberships, and certifications. Unlike a resume, a CV continues to grow throughout your career.

Most nurses applying to nurse anesthesiology school do not yet have an academic CV—and that is perfectly appropriate. If you already have a CV, you may certainly submit it unless the program requests a resume. However, if you do not have a CV, **do not create one simply for your application.** A well-organized resume is more than sufficient and is often easier for admissions committees to review quickly.

Whether you submit a resume or a CV, your document should be organized, concise, and easy to navigate.

Your Resume May Be Reviewed by More Than People

As artificial intelligence becomes increasingly integrated into higher education, portions of your application may be reviewed electronically before a faculty member ever sees it.

Many universities use a cloud-based customer relationship management (CRM) platform, such as **Salesforce**, to organize and manage applications. In nursing education, many programs also utilize **NursingCAS**, the centralized application service operated by the American Association of Colleges of Nursing (AACN).

NursingCAS serves as the front-end application portal for applicants, while platforms such as Salesforce often serve as the back-end system used by admissions offices to organize and review applications. Some schools use both systems, while others use only one or use entirely different platforms.

Because every institution uses different software, applicants rarely know exactly how their materials will be processed. Some applications may receive AI-assisted screening, while others may be reviewed exclusively by faculty. The important takeaway is this: create a clean, organized resume that is easy for both people and technology to understand.

What Are We Looking For On Your Resume?

As a program director, I review approximately 500 applications each year. During peak admission season, I often spend one minute—or less—reviewing each resume before deciding whether to continue exploring an applicant's file.

When I open your resume, I want to quickly find the answers to several questions:

- What is your highest degree earned and is your GPA listed (If not, why not?)
- What professional licenses and specialty certifications do you hold? Specifically, did you obtain your CCRN?
- Where did you complete your education?
- How many years have you worked in healthcare?
- How many years have you worked specifically as a critical care nurse?
- What critical care units have you worked in?
- What leadership roles have you held?
- Have you ever precepted in the ICU?
- What committees, quality improvement projects, or research have you participated in?
- Have you shadowed a CRNA or anesthesiologist? If so, where and for how many hours?

- What accomplishments distinguish you from other applicants?

If I must search for these answers, your resume is working against you.

Highlight Specialized Skills

Don't overlook specialized skills that are directly applicable to nurse anesthesiology. One of the most important examples is ultrasound. Ultrasound has become an indispensable tool in modern anesthesia practice. It is routinely used for vascular access, regional anesthesia, and point-of-care assessment.

If you have been trained in ultrasound-guided peripheral IV placement or have experience using ultrasound in your current practice, be sure that it is clearly listed on your resume.

This is not a skill every ICU nurse possesses, and it immediately demonstrates experience with technology that you will continue to use throughout your nurse anesthesiology education and career. Rather than burying it within a job description, list it as a technical proficiency so it is easy for reviewers to find.

Organizing Your Credentials

One of the first things admissions committees notice is how you present your professional credentials.

The order of credentials varies somewhat by state and employer, but a commonly accepted sequence recommended by professional nursing organizations is:

Highest academic degree → Professional license → Specialty certifications

Examples include:

- Jamie Doe, BSN, RN, CCRN
- Jessie Doe, MSN, RN
- Alex Smith, DNP, APRN, CRNA

Avoid listing credentials that are expired or no longer applicable and ensure that every certification listed is current.

Do not list your life support classes or a specialty course you took.

For most nurse anesthesiology program applications, simplicity is best. If you have earned multiple nursing degrees, it is generally sufficient to list only your highest nursing degree with your name.

For example, if you earned a BSN and later completed an MSN, listing **MSN, RN** is appropriate. Your BSN should still appear in the education section of your resume or CV, but it does not need to be included in your credential line.

Likewise, degrees earned outside of nursing should be included in the education section of your resume but generally do not need to appear with your professional credentials. For example, an applicant who has earned a Master of Business Administration (MBA) should certainly list that degree in the education section, but it is usually unnecessary to include **MBA** after their name when applying to a nurse anesthesiology program. A cleaner presentation would be:

Alex Smith, MSN, RN, CCRN

rather than

Alex Smith, MSN, RN, CCRN, MBA

The goal is not to minimize your accomplishments but to emphasize the credentials that are most relevant to your role as a critical care nurse and future nurse anesthesiologist.

A well-organized resume does more than list your accomplishments—it makes it easy for admissions committees to recognize your qualifications within seconds. Your goal is not to impress reviewers with the length of your document, but with the clarity of your professional journey.

Anesthesia Shadowing

When I was in anesthesia school, I had a classmate who stepped into an operating room for the very first time during our initial clinical rotation. Within a short period, she began developing persistent headaches whenever she was in the perioperative environment. It was never clear whether they were caused by trace anesthetic gases, surgical smoke, disinfectants, or another environmental exposure. Despite trying to push through, the symptoms persisted. About six months into the program, she made the difficult decision to withdraw in order to protect her health.

That experience has stayed with me throughout my career.

As a program director, one of my greatest responsibilities is admitting students who have the greatest likelihood of successfully completing the program. Nurse anesthesiology education is demanding for students, faculty, clinical partners, and universities alike. Students invest years of preparation, leave careers, relocate families, and often assume significant educational debt. Programs commit substantial faculty time and limited clinical training resources. When a student discovers after admission that the operating room is simply not the right environment for them, everyone loses.

For that reason, I have a personal policy that I will not advocate for admitting an applicant who has never spent meaningful time observing in the operating room. Shadowing is not simply a box to check on an application—it is an opportunity to answer one important question:

Can I truly see myself doing this work every day?

The operating room is unlike any other healthcare environment. It has its own culture, pace, sounds, smells, personalities, and expectations. Some people immediately feel at home. Others quickly realize it is not where they thrive. Both outcomes are valuable because it is far better to discover that before beginning a three-year doctoral program than six months into one.

I encourage every prospective applicant to shadow multiple CRNAs whenever possible. Observe different types of cases, different facilities, and different practice settings. Ask questions. Watch how the CRNA interacts with surgeons, nurses, anesthesia technicians, and, most importantly, patients.

Remember that once you graduate, you may ultimately practice in virtually any environment where CRNAs are employed. You may choose an Anesthesia Care Team (ACT) practice, where anesthesiologists and CRNAs collaborate, or an independent practice setting in which CRNAs provide anesthesia care autonomously. If possible, observe both models. Not only will they help you determine whether nurse anesthesiology is the right profession for you, but they may also influence the type of practice you hope to pursue after graduation.

One challenge applicants face today is that shadowing opportunities have become increasingly difficult to obtain. Many hospitals and surgery centers have implemented stricter policies regarding observers because of privacy regulations, infection prevention practices, liability concerns, and administrative requirements. As a result, simply calling an operating room and asking to shadow is often no longer enough.

This is where professional relationships become incredibly valuable. Reach out to CRNAs you know through work, school, professional organizations, former classmates, friends, or colleagues. Be respectful of their time, remain flexible with scheduling, and recognize that arranging a shadowing experience often requires someone to advocate for you behind the scenes.

As an admissions committee member, I recognize the effort it takes to secure these opportunities. When I see applicants who have shadowed at multiple facilities or with several different CRNAs, I am genuinely impressed. It tells me they were willing to invest the time, build relationships, and seek out a broader understanding of the profession rather than settling for the minimum. Those experiences almost always lead to richer interview conversations because the applicant has seen nurse anesthesiology practiced in a variety of environments.

Make the Most of Your Shadowing Experience

Many applicants think shadowing means quietly standing in the corner of the operating room. While there are certainly times when you simply need to observe, shadowing should be an active learning experience. A CRNA who has agreed to let you spend the day with them is usually happy to answer questions when it is appropriate and safe to do so.

Instead of focusing only on the technical procedures, try to understand the clinical reasoning behind what you are seeing. Consider asking questions such as:

- Why did you choose this anesthetic technique instead of another?
- What factors influenced your airway assessment and airway plan?
- What are you watching most closely on the monitors right now?
- Why did you choose this vasoactive medication instead of a different one?
- What complications are you anticipating for this patient?
- How do you decide when a patient is ready for emergence?
- What aspects of your job do you enjoy the most?
- What are the biggest challenges of being a CRNA?

- If you could go back, would you choose this profession again?

You should also pay attention to things that have nothing to do with pharmacology or physiology. Watch how the CRNA communicates with anxious patients before surgery. Observe how they collaborate with surgeons, nurses, anesthesia technicians, and anesthesiologists. Notice how they remain calm when unexpected situations arise. These professional behaviors are just as important as the technical aspects of anesthesia practice.

Finally, pay attention to yourself. Can you picture yourself in this environment every day? Does the pace energize you? Do you enjoy solving problems in real time? Can you see yourself comforting patients who are often experiencing one of the most stressful moments of their lives? Those answers are every bit as important as anything you learn about anesthetic drugs or airway management.

If, after several shadowing experiences, you find yourself excited to return to the operating room, you have learned something incredibly important. If you realize it is not the right fit, that is equally valuable. Our healthcare system needs exceptional nurses in every specialty, and I am genuinely grateful for those who determine that becoming a CRNA is not their path.

Either way, shadowing is one of the least expensive and most informative investments you can make before applying to nurse anesthesiology school.

One additional piece of advice: even if you have worked in the operating room, do not list that experience as "shadowing" on your application or résumé.

I once interviewed an applicant who proudly presented a spreadsheet documenting more than 400 hours of anesthesia shadowing. Naturally, I was impressed and asked how she had accumulated so many hours. She explained that she had previously worked as a circulating operating room nurse and had counted her work hours as shadowing.

That is not shadowing—it is employment.

Ironically, her operating room experience was a genuine strength, but presenting it as shadowing made her appear disingenuous. It raised unnecessary questions about her judgment and credibility during an interview where honesty matters immensely.

Programs ask about shadowing because we want to know that you intentionally spent time observing a CRNA in the anesthesia role.

Shadowing means following the CRNA through the entire patient experience—from the preoperative assessment and anesthetic plan, to induction, maintenance, emergence, postoperative handoff, and the countless clinical decisions made throughout the case. It is a deliberate educational experience, not simply being present in the operating room as part of another job.

If you have operating room experience, absolutely highlight it. It demonstrates familiarity with the perioperative environment and is often a significant strength in your application. Just present it accurately. List your operating room employment as employment and your CRNA shadowing as shadowing. Admissions committees value both, but they are not the same thing.

One final thought: quality matters far more than quantity. I would rather interview an applicant who spent twenty thoughtful hours actively engaged with a CRNA than someone who logged one hundred hours while staring at the anesthesia machine. Shadowing is not about accumulating hours—it is about gaining perspective. If you leave the operating room with a clearer understanding of the profession and even greater enthusiasm for becoming a CRNA, then you have accomplished exactly what shadowing is intended to do.

The Good Resume

The resume on the next page is an example of the format I encourage applicants to use. My philosophy is simple: include the information that matters most and leave out what admissions committees already know. This resume is not for the faint of heart. I am going to ask you to whittle your document down to the most minimal terminology possible. As I have mentioned, I do not have the time to complete a word find when I read your resume. If I cannot find what I am looking for, I will quickly move on. Make it easy for us Program Directors.

Furthermore, please remember that the people reviewing your application are experienced ICU nurses, CRNAs, and anesthesia faculty. You do not need to explain that you can titrate vasoactive medications, provide compassionate care, or perform the routine responsibilities expected of every critical care nurse. Those are baseline expectations, and your ability to demonstrate them will be evaluated during the interview.

Instead, be concise and intentional. Every line on your resume should tell the reader something meaningful about you—your accomplishments, leadership, specialized skills, certifications, and professional growth.

Perhaps most importantly, a focused resume demonstrates respect for your audience. By avoiding a lengthy ICU job description, you acknowledge that the reader already understands what an experienced critical care nurse does. That subtle professionalism makes a strong impression and helps your application stand out for the right reasons.

Side note: You do not need to include a headshot, color blocking, or your home address. Your name, credentials, phone number, and email are all that are needed.

Matthew J. Frost, BSN, RN, CCRN

612-555-1122 m_frost@gmail.com

EDUCATION

University of Wisconsin – Eau Claire — Eau Claire, WI
Bachelor of Science – Nursing — June 2023

- GPA 3.5
- Cum Laude

Chippewa Valley Technical College — Eau Claire, WI
Associate's Degree – Nursing — May 2021

- GPA 3.6
- President's List
- Honors Student

WORK EXPERIENCE

Registered Nurse — Rochester, MN
Mayo Clinic Health System CVICU — June 2023 - Current

- 3.5 years Critical Care Experience
- Co-Chair Professional Development Committee
- Preceptor
- Proficiencies: LVAD, CRRT, ECMO, Post-op hearts
- Ultrasound-guided peripheral IV insertion

Registered Nurse — Eau Claire, WI
HSHS Sacred Heart Hospital Med Surg — June 2021 – Aug. 2022

- 1 year of experience

LICENSES & CERTIFICATIONS

Registered Nurse – State of Minnesota

CCRN

ACLS, PALS, BLS

Trauma Nursing Core Course

ANESTHESIA SHADOWING

Mayo Clinic Health System — 2025 & 2026

- 16 + Hours CRNA Shadowing

There are many ways to write an excellent resume. This example is not the only correct format, but it illustrates many of the characteristics I appreciate when reviewing applications.

As a program director, I am looking at multiple resume's and trying to glean the information I need to know. The more clean and easy to read a resume, the more positive I feel towards the candidate. During application season, I simply do not have the luxury of reading lengthy descriptions of every applicant's responsibilities. My goal is to determine, as efficiently as possible, whether you possess the experience, knowledge, and skills necessary to be successful in nurse anesthesiology school.

This resume accomplishes exactly that.

It tells me who you are immediately.

Within the first few seconds, I know the applicant's highest nursing degree, nursing license, and specialty certification. There is no guessing and no searching.

It shows me your educational journey.

The education section is concise but complete. I can quickly see where the applicant attended school, when degrees were earned, academic achievements, and GPA.

It focuses on accomplishments rather than job descriptions.

One of the biggest mistakes applicants make is copying and pasting their hospital job description into their resume. I don't need to know that you "provide patient-centered care," "administer medications," or "collaborate with the interdisciplinary team." Every ICU nurse does those things.

Instead, I want to know what makes **you** different.

Tell me that you are a preceptor. Tell me you chair a committee. Tell me you have experience with ECMO, CRRT, LVADs, ventricular assist devices, post-operative cardiac surgery, or ultrasound-guided IV placement. Those are the details that help me understand the complexity of your practice.

It tells me your experience at a glance.

One of my favorite features of this resume is that it clearly states the applicant's total critical care experience.

I should not have to calculate dates in my head to determine how long you have been a nurse or how much ICU experience you have. Make it easy for the admissions committee.

Likewise, if you worked in another nursing specialty before transferring to critical care, let me know how many years you spent in each role.

It emphasizes skills instead of hospital reputation.

Applicants sometimes worry because they work at a hospital I may not recognize or in an ICU located outside of Minnesota.

That doesn't concern me nearly as much as you might think.

I may not know exactly how your unit operates, but I do want to know what you are capable of doing. Describe your patient population (i.e. Cardiovascular ICU) and the advanced therapies you routinely manage. Those skills tell me far more than the hospital's name ever could.

It includes the information I care about.

Notice that this resume clearly lists licenses, certifications, committee involvement, technical proficiencies, and anesthesia shadowing experience. These are all important pieces of information that help paint a picture of the applicant's readiness for nurse anesthesiology school.

It avoids unnecessary distractions.

This resume uses a simple, clean layout without photographs, graphics, colored boxes, icons, or elaborate formatting. While those design elements may look attractive, they rarely add value to a graduate school application and can actually make important information more difficult to find. Remember that your goal is clarity—not decoration.

It becomes a useful interview tool.

Perhaps my favorite quality of this resume is that it naturally guides the interview.

When I review this document, I immediately know what I want to ask about. I can ask about the applicant's committee leadership, ECMO experience, ultrasound-guided IV skills, or shadowing experiences. The resume creates meaningful conversation because it highlights the experiences that truly distinguish the applicant.

Applicants often ask me whether they should have a one-page resume. My answer is yes. If you have additional leadership experience, volunteer work, research, presentations, or publications, absolutely include them. However, recognize that the first page is your first impression. If I can understand who you are and what you bring to the profession within the first minute, you've created a resume that works for you instead of against you.

What About Volunteer Experience?

One question I am occasionally asked is whether volunteer experience is necessary to be a competitive nurse anesthesiology applicant.

My answer may surprise you.

Unlike applicants to medical school or physician assistant programs, nurse anesthesiology applicants are already experienced healthcare professionals. By the time you apply, you have likely spent years caring for critically ill patients on nights, weekends, holidays, and in some of the most emotionally demanding situations imaginable.

Every shift requires compassion, service, teamwork, and sacrifice. In many ways, your career as an ICU nurse is already a life of service.

For that reason, I have never placed significant weight on volunteer hours during the admissions process. In all my years reviewing applications, I have never looked at an otherwise strong candidate and thought, "If only they had volunteered another 100 hours."

Instead, I focus on the qualities that have consistently predicted success in nurse anesthesiology school: strong academics, meaningful ICU experience, critical thinking, professionalism, leadership, communication skills, emotional maturity, and a genuine commitment to lifelong learning.

That does **not** mean volunteer work is unimportant. If serving your community is something you genuinely enjoy and have done consistently over time, absolutely include it on your resume. Long-term service that reflects your passions and values helps tell the story of who you are as a person. Authenticity is always more meaningful than checking a box.

What I do **not** recommend is taking on volunteer commitments solely because you think they will make your application more competitive.

As nurses, we sometimes feel guilty saying no. We are caregivers by nature, and we often believe that doing more is always better. But I would encourage you to think differently.

Critical care nursing is demanding. Many of you are balancing full-time work, night shifts, overtime, professional certifications, continuing education, family responsibilities, and preparing your graduate school application. Your time away from work is valuable. It is okay—healthy, even—to use that time to recharge.

Spend time with your spouse or partner. Be present for your children. Exercise. Travel. Read. Developing hobbies. Get enough sleep. Protect your physical and mental health. Those experiences are not wasted time; they build the resilience that will carry you through the challenges of nurse anesthesiology school and your future career.

One of the most important lessons you can learn before graduate school is that taking care of yourself is not selfish—it is professional. The best clinicians recognize that they cannot provide exceptional care for others if they continually neglect themselves.

Throughout this book, I have encouraged you to avoid chasing résumé checkboxes and instead focus on becoming the kind of clinician who naturally stands out. This is another example of that philosophy. Build a career, a character, and a life that reflect your values. If volunteer service is genuinely part of that story, it belongs on your resume. If it is something you feel pressured to add simply to impress an admissions committee, your energy is probably better invested elsewhere.

What about Life Support Certifications?

One of the questions I hear frequently is whether applicants should obtain every possible life support certification before applying to nurse anesthesiology school.

My advice is simple: don't spend money on certifications you do not yet need. However, any school could want the certifications at any time. Your best bet is to ask the admissions office if you need to have all of the certifications or not before you apply.

You will need current life support certifications when you begin your clinical education. Those certifications must remain current throughout your clinical training and, in many cases, until you have successfully passed the National Certification Examination (NCE). However, most programs do **not** require every certification before you even start school.

For example, if you currently work exclusively with adult patients, there is usually little benefit to obtaining your Pediatric Advanced Life Support (PALS) certification before admission. You will have plenty of time to complete it before you begin caring for pediatric patients during your clinical rotations. Admissions committees understand this. We would rather see you save your money and obtain certifications when they are actually needed than spend hundreds of dollars trying to make your application appear stronger.

The same principle applies to other certifications. If a certification is directly applicable to your current role, it is often worthwhile. If you are obtaining it solely because you think it will impress an admissions committee, it probably is not the best investment of your time or money.

One recommendation I do make is to obtain your certifications through the **American Heart Association (AHA)** whenever possible. The AHA remains the gold standard for Basic Life Support (BLS), Advanced Cardiovascular Life Support (ACLS), and Pediatric Advanced Life Support (PALS). While some organizations offer equivalent courses, many hospitals, universities, and clinical affiliates specifically require AHA certification. Completing an AHA course from the beginning can prevent unnecessary inconvenience later.

Finally, always verify the requirements of the programs to which you are applying. Schools and clinical affiliates occasionally have different expectations regarding acceptable providers, expiration dates, and required certifications. A quick email or phone call before registering for a course can save you both time and money.

Life support certifications are important, but they are not what gets you admitted. Strong clinical experience, excellent academic preparation, thoughtful shadowing, and professionalism will have a much greater impact on your application than collecting certifications you may not need yet.

Nursing License

An unencumbered registered nursing license is required before you can begin a nurse anesthesiology program. Throughout your education, you will be providing patient care under your own nursing license, so maintaining an active license in good standing is essential.

As part of our admissions process at Saint Mary's, we ask applicants whether they hold a Minnesota Registered Nurse license. You do **not** need to have a Minnesota license at the time you apply, but you will need one before the program begins. Keep in mind that Minnesota is **not** a member of the Nurse Licensure Compact (NLC), so a multistate license from another compact state does not authorize you to practice in Minnesota. Every program has its own licensure requirements, so be sure to review the school's website carefully to determine which state license is required before classes and clinical experiences begin.

Just as with life support certifications, avoid making assumptions based on another school's requirements. Verify exactly what your program expects before spending time and money obtaining additional licenses or credentials.

One piece of advice I cannot emphasize enough is this: **protect your nursing license.** It is your livelihood, and it is the foundation upon which your anesthesia career will be built.

I once had a student begin the program and then disclose that she was under investigation by her state Board of Nursing because of a medication error. It was a heartbreaking situation. Everyone involved understood that if her nursing license were suspended or revoked, she would no longer be eligible to continue in the program. The uncertainty alone created enormous stress during an already demanding educational experience.

Mistakes happen in healthcare, and Boards of Nursing recognize that. However, honesty and transparency are always the best approach. If you have a current Board investigation, disciplinary action, or another issue that could affect your nursing license, discuss it with the program before you enroll. It is far better to have an honest conversation upfront than to create a situation that jeopardizes your education after you have already invested significant time, money, and effort.

Your nursing license is one of your most valuable professional assets. Guard it carefully.

A Real-World Good Resume Example

This advice isn't limited to graduate school applications. Although multiple nurses have taken my resume guidance and successfully got into a nurse anesthesiology program, I have an example from the employment side, too.

A few years ago, my husband, who is also a registered nurse, decided to apply for a highly sought-after remote nursing position within his healthcare organization. The role involved providing telephone triage and patient support from home.

My husband's employer employs nearly 500 nurses, and these positions are extremely competitive. Approximately 50 nurses typically apply each time an opening becomes available.

He had worked for the organization for eight years, so the hiring managers already understood what bedside nurses do. They didn't need another resume filled with generic nursing responsibilities. Instead, we created a simple, organized resume that highlighted his credentials, years of experience, leadership activities, certifications, and the skills that made him stand out from the other applicants.

He was offered an interview and ultimately received the position.

Afterward, the hiring team specifically commented on how much they appreciated the format of his resume. They told him they were able to find exactly what they needed without sorting through paragraphs of unnecessary information.

That experience reinforced something I have learned after reviewing hundreds of graduate school applications: whether you are applying for a nurse anesthesiology program or a nursing position, your resume should make the reviewer's job easier—not harder. The easier it is to understand your qualifications, the more likely they are to remember you.

Bring Your Resume to the Interview

As I hinted at earlier, once you've created a polished resume, don't leave it at home.

Bring several high-quality printed copies of your resume to every program interview, even if you previously uploaded it as part of your application. Interviewers may have reviewed your file weeks or even months earlier, and not everyone on the interview panel will necessarily have a copy in front of them.

At the beginning of the interview, offer a copy to each interviewer. It is a simple professional courtesy that demonstrates preparation and attention to detail. More importantly, it gives the interviewers a roadmap for your conversation. A well-organized resume allows them to quickly reference your experiences, ask meaningful questions about your leadership, committee work, certifications, and specialized skills, and spend less time searching through your application. Your resume should work for you throughout the interview, serving as a concise summary of your professional journey and helping guide the discussion toward the experiences that make you a strong future nurse anesthesiologist.

Reflection Questions

1. If an admissions committee spent only 30 seconds reviewing my resume, what three things would I want them to remember about me?
2. Does my resume tell the story of who I am as a critical care nurse, or does it simply list where I have worked?
3. What experiences, certifications, leadership roles, committee work, or volunteer activities demonstrate that I have gone beyond the minimum expectations of my position?
4. Have I highlighted the skills that are most relevant to nurse anesthesiology, such as charge nurse experience, precepting, CCRN certification, ultrasound-guided IV placement, rapid response participation, or ECMO, CRRT, and other advanced critical care experience?
5. Is my resume organized in a way that makes it easy for an admissions committee to quickly identify my strengths?
6. If I were interviewing tomorrow, would I be proud to hand my resume to every person on the interview panel?
7. Looking at my resume today, what one addition or improvement would make me a stronger applicant over the next year?

Specialty Certifications: What should I consider?

One credential that many nurse anesthesiology programs either require or strongly recommend is the Critical Care Registered Nurse (CCRN) certification. While the CCRN certainly demonstrates advanced knowledge of critical care nursing, its value in the admissions process extends well beyond the letters after your name. Simply put, the CCRN tells admissions committees two important things. First, it confirms that you have spent enough time in the intensive care unit to develop the depth of clinical experience expected of a future nurse anesthetist. You cannot successfully earn the CCRN without meaningful bedside critical care experience. Second, it demonstrates that you are willing and able to dedicate yourself to studying for—and successfully passing—a rigorous professional certification exam. Graduate school in nurse anesthesiology requires discipline, perseverance, and the ability to master large amounts of complex information. Successfully preparing for the CCRN provides evidence that you possess those qualities before you ever submit your application.

As a program director, I often tell prospective students that the CCRN is about much more than critical care knowledge. It is evidence that you have invested in yourself professionally, challenged yourself academically, and followed through on a difficult goal. If I am reviewing two applicants with similar academic records, comparable ICU experience, and strong interviews, but only one has taken the initiative to earn the CCRN, that certification becomes another piece of evidence that the applicant is committed to excellence. It tells me they were willing to do the hard work before graduate school even began. While the CCRN alone will not guarantee admission, it is one of the clearest ways to demonstrate both clinical maturity and readiness for the academic rigor of nurse anesthesiology education.

One reason the CCRN carries so much weight is that nurse anesthesiology programs do not have a standardized entrance examination that allows admissions committees to compare applicants using a single objective measure. Medical schools have the MCAT, law schools have the LSAT, and many graduate programs have historically relied on the GRE. Nurse anesthesiology education has no equivalent exam. Instead, admissions committees must evaluate academic readiness by looking at the totality of an applicant's record: undergraduate and graduate coursework, science performance, ICU experience, professional recommendations, interviews, and specialty certifications.

The CCRN has become one of the most valuable of these credentials because it is nationally recognized, academically rigorous, and directly relevant to critical care practice. While it is not a perfect substitute for a standardized entrance examination, it provides admissions committees with additional confidence that an applicant has both the knowledge base and the study habits necessary to succeed in one of the most academically demanding nursing specialties.

For applicants, my advice is simple: if you meet the eligibility requirements, earn your CCRN before you apply. It strengthens your application, deepens your critical care knowledge, and demonstrates a level of professional commitment that admissions committees notice. More importantly, the knowledge and study habits you develop while preparing for the exam will continue to serve you well throughout nurse anesthesiology school and beyond.

What is the CCRN?

The **CCRN® exam** is the American Association of Critical-Care Nurses' (AACN) professional certification exam for nurses who provide direct care to acutely and critically ill patients.
Here's a detailed breakdown:

Purpose

To validate that you have the advanced clinical knowledge and judgment necessary to care for patients with complex, life-threatening conditions in intensive care or specialty units.

Eligibility

You must be an RN or APRN with:

- **Option 1**: At least **1,750 hours** of direct care for acutely/critically ill patients in the past 2 years, with **875 of those hours** in the most recent year.
- **Option 2**: At least **2,000 hours** in the past 5 years, with **144 of those hours** in the most recent year.
- Hours can be in adult, pediatric, or neonatal critical care (you choose the population when applying).

Format

- **Computer-based exam** at a testing center or live remote proctoring.
- **Length**: 3 hours
- **Questions**: 150 multiple-choice questions
    - 125 scored

    - 25 unscored (pilot questions that don't count toward your score)

- **Passing score**: Scaled score of **83** out of 125 scored questions (AACN doesn't publish raw % thresholds, but this is roughly 66%).

Content Outline

The CCRN exam tests *two domains*: **Clinical Judgment** and **Professional Caring & Ethical Practice**.

A. Clinical Judgment (80% of exam)

Organized by body systems:

- **Cardiovascular** – ~17%
- **Pulmonary** – ~15%
- **Endocrine/Hematology/Gastrointestinal/Renal/Integumentary** – ~20% combined
- **Multisystem** (shock, sepsis, trauma, burns) – ~14%
- **Neurology** – ~10%
- **Behavioral/Psychosocial** – ~5%

B. Professional Caring & Ethical Practice (20% of exam)

Covers:

- Advocacy & moral agency
- Caring practices
- Collaboration
- Systems thinking
- Response to diversity
- Clinical inquiry

Question Style

- Scenario-based critical thinking questions
- Requires interpreting labs, hemodynamic data, ECG strips, and ventilator settings
- Often asks: *"What is the BEST next step?"* rather than simple recall

CCRN Pass Rate

As of January 2026, The national pass rate of the Adult CCRN exam is about 79%, with the neonatal and pediatric pass rates coming in at 67% and 76%, respectively. A candidate can take it up to four times in a 12 month period. This pass rate demonstrates that the exam is rigorous, and that not all individuals are able to pass it on the first try. It certainly gives program directors reassurance that you must prepare and apply yourself in order to pass the exam.

CFRN

If you are a flight nurse, earning the Certified Flight Registered Nurse (CFRN) credential is an excellent way to demonstrate your clinical expertise and professional commitment. Like the CCRN, the CFRN requires extensive preparation and successful completion of a rigorous national certification examination. It signals to admissions committees that you have challenged yourself academically and have developed advanced critical thinking skills while caring for critically ill patients in complex environments. Although the CCRN remains the certification most closely aligned with the knowledge and experience expected of ICU nurses entering nurse anesthesiology school, the CFRN is equally respected for applicants whose primary practice is flight or critical care transport. Ultimately, the strongest certification is the one that best reflects your clinical role and demonstrates your commitment to professional excellence.

Who is the CFRN for?

- Registered nurses who provide care in air medical transport (helicopter or fixed-wing aircraft) or other critical care transport settings.

What does it demonstrate?

- Advanced knowledge of emergency medicine, critical care, trauma, transport physiology, and the care of critically ill patients outside the traditional hospital environment.

Why is it valuable?

- The CFRN is a nationally recognized board certification that demonstrates clinical expertise, critical thinking, and a commitment to professional development. Like the CCRN, it requires dedicated preparation and successful completion of a challenging certification examination.

How do admissions committees view it?

- The CFRN is highly respected by nurse anesthesiology programs, particularly for applicants whose primary clinical practice is flight or critical care transport. While the CCRN remains the certification most closely aligned with traditional ICU nursing, the CFRN provides comparable evidence of academic preparation, professional dedication, and advanced clinical judgment.

TNCC

Another certification many critical care nurses pursue is the Trauma Nursing Core Course (TNCC). The TNCC is an outstanding educational program that enhances the assessment and management of injured patients and is especially valuable for nurses working in trauma centers or emergency departments. However, from an admissions perspective, we generally place greater emphasis on the CCRN. Unlike the TNCC, which is primarily an educational course focused on trauma care, the CCRN is a nationally recognized certification examination that validates comprehensive critical care knowledge gained through extensive bedside ICU experience.

The CCRN also requires a significant commitment to independent study and mastery of complex critical care concepts. For those reasons, it provides admissions committees with stronger evidence of both clinical expertise and academic readiness. If you have both certifications, that's wonderful—but if you are deciding where to invest your time and energy before applying to nurse anesthesiology school, I would encourage you to prioritize earning your CCRN.

What is the TNCC?

TNCC — Trauma Nursing Core Course

- **Type**: Course certification (not a professional credential)
- **Purpose**: Teaches a standardized, systematic approach to caring for trauma patients in the **first hours** after injury.
- **Audience**: Primarily ER, trauma, flight, and critical care nurses who may respond to trauma cases.
- **Focus**:
    - Initial trauma assessment (primary/secondary survey)
    - Airway, breathing, circulation priorities
    - Rapid stabilization techniques
    - Mechanisms of injury & special populations (peds, burns, etc.)
- **Administered by**: Emergency Nurses Association (ENA)
- **Format**: 2-day course with lecture, skills stations, and written/practical tests

- **Validity**: Typically 4 years, then recertification required

Think of TNCC as *training in a trauma response protocol* — similar to ACLS or PALS but for trauma.

Other Critical Care Credentials

In addition to the CCRN and CFRN, there are several other specialty credentials that may strengthen your professional profile depending on your role and practice setting.

Certified Transport Registered Nurse (CTRN)

Designed for nurses who provide ground critical care transport, the CTRN demonstrates expertise in the care and transport of critically ill and injured patients. It is a respected credential for nurses whose primary practice is mobile critical care.

CCRN-K

The CCRN-K is intended for experienced critical care nurses who have transitioned away from direct bedside care into leadership, education, research, or other advanced professional roles. Rather than focusing on hands-on patient care, it recognizes continued expertise and contributions to the specialty of critical care nursing.

Progressive Care Certified Nurse (PCCN)

The PCCN is designed for nurses who care for acutely ill adult patients in progressive care, step-down, telemetry, or intermediate care units. While it is a valuable certification for nurses practicing in those settings, it generally does not carry the same weight as the CCRN for applicants to nurse anesthesiology programs because it reflects a lower-acuity patient population than the intensive care unit.

As you can see, there are many opportunities to grow professionally as a critical care nurse. Whether you choose to earn the CCRN, CFRN, CTRN, TNCC, or another specialty credential, each represents an investment in your knowledge and your patients. From an admissions standpoint, however, the certifications that carry the greatest weight are those that demonstrate both advanced critical care expertise and the discipline required to prepare for a rigorous national examination. Remember, our goal is not simply to admit applicants with impressive resumes—we are looking for future colleagues who have already developed a habit of lifelong learning. Every certification you earn, every course you complete, and every challenge you choose to undertake tells us something about your commitment to excellence. That commitment will serve you well not only during the admissions process but throughout your career as a nurse anesthesiologist.

Reflection Questions:

1. Which specialty certification best aligns with my current clinical role, and what steps can I take to earn it before I apply?
2. If I am eligible for the CCRN, what has prevented me from taking the exam? Is it lack of time, confidence, or commitment?
3. How would earning a specialty certification strengthen not only my application but also my confidence as a critical care nurse?
4. Beyond meeting minimum requirements, what evidence can I provide that demonstrates my commitment to lifelong learning?
5. If I were sitting on an admissions committee, what would my current certifications say about my professional growth and readiness for graduate education?
6. What is one professional goal I can accomplish in the next six months that will make me a stronger nurse anesthesiology applicant?
7. Am I pursuing certifications because they will improve my résumé, or because they will make me a better clinician? How can I ensure those goals remain connected?

8. Looking at my application as a whole, where are my strengths and where could additional professional development help me stand out?

GPA: Demonstrating Your Academic Readiness

For many applicants, GPA is one of the most stressful parts of the application process. Unfortunately, there is no universal entrance exam for nurse anesthesiology programs that allows applicants to demonstrate academic ability on a level playing field. As a result, admissions committees often rely heavily on your academic record to help assess your readiness for the rigorous curriculum.

Some programs may go beyond your transcript by asking clinically focused interview questions or requiring written responses that help assess your knowledge, critical thinking, and clinical judgment. With more than 150 nurse anesthesiology programs across the country, every admissions process is a little different, so it is impossible to predict exactly how each school will evaluate applicants. What I can do is offer some practical guidance on how to think about your GPA.

If your GPA is not where you would like it to be, remember that you cannot change the grades you have already earned—but you can influence how your academic record looks moving forward. One option is to retake courses, when permitted, to demonstrate improved academic performance. Another option is to pursue additional graduate-level coursework or even complete a master's degree in nursing before applying. Strong performance in recent, rigorous coursework can help demonstrate that you are academically prepared for doctoral education.

Before investing significant time and money into additional classes or another degree, take the time to calculate how those new grades would affect your overall GPA and your science GPA. In some cases, a few carefully selected courses can make a meaningful difference. In other situations, the improvement may be modest despite a substantial investment. Understanding the potential impact beforehand will help you make informed decisions about where to spend your time, effort, and resources.

This is a challenge faced by many applicants, and it often leads to a difficult question: *Do I continue working intentionally to strengthen my GPA in hopes of gaining admission, or is it time to consider a different career path?* There is no right or wrong answer. Only you can decide whether the investment of time, money, and energy aligns with your personal and professional goals.

I have had many conversations with applicants in this position. My advice is usually the same: there is nothing wrong with applying, but it is important to be realistic about the competitiveness of the applicant pool. Across the country, GPA remains one of the strongest predictors used to determine who receives an interview. Applying may help you understand where you stand, but it should also be accompanied by an honest assessment of whether your application is as competitive as it could be.

When I recommend additional education, I am often referring to a graduate degree such as a leadership-focused Master of Science in Nursing (MSN). Graduate-level coursework completed with excellent grades can strengthen your cumulative GPA while also demonstrating your ability to succeed in advanced academic work. Before enrolling, however, calculate the potential impact. Completing twenty graduate credits with A's may meaningfully improve one applicant's GPA while having only a modest effect for another.

One of the hardest parts of being a program director is balancing encouragement with honesty. Every admissions committee wants to admit applicants who are compassionate, clinically skilled, and deeply committed to becoming CRNAs. But we also have an obligation to admit students who have demonstrated the academic preparation needed to succeed in one of the most demanding graduate programs in nursing. That responsibility extends beyond admission. It includes helping ensure that students are ultimately successful on the National Certification Examination and enter practice as safe, competent providers.

Over the years, I have known remarkable nurses who possessed outstanding clinical judgment, exceptional work ethic, and all the personal qualities needed to become excellent CRNAs. Unfortunately, some struggled with the academic intensity of nurse anesthesiology education and were ultimately unable to complete the program or pass boards. Watching someone accumulate significant educational debt without achieving the career they dreamed of is heartbreaking.

That is why I believe applicants deserve honesty. My goal is never to discourage you. It is to help you make the most informed decision possible. If strengthening your academic record gives you a realistic path toward admission, then I encourage you to pursue it with purpose. If, after careful consideration, another path seems more appropriate, know that there are countless meaningful ways to make an extraordinary impact as a nurse. Success is not defined by becoming a CRNA—it is defined by finding the role where your talents, passions, and preparation come together to serve others well.

Calculating Your Science and Math GPA

One of the first exercises I recommend to every applicant is calculating your science and math GPA. While every program has its own method for evaluating transcripts, many schools place particular emphasis on your performance in science, mathematics, and nursing coursework because these subjects most closely reflect the academic demands of nurse anesthesiology education.

The Science and Math GPA worksheet is the one currently used by the Saint Mary's University of Minnesota Nurse Anesthesiology Admissions Committee to calculate an applicant's science and math GPA. Although other programs may use different criteria, this worksheet provides a practical example of how an admissions committee may evaluate your academic record.

Completing the science and math worksheet (Appendix A) can help you identify your academic strengths, recognize areas that could be improved, and estimate how additional coursework or repeated classes might influence your GPA before investing additional time and money. Even if you are not applying to Saint Mary's, I encourage you to perform this calculation. Understanding your academic profile is one of the most valuable steps you can take as you prepare your application.

Reflection Questions

1. Have I taken an honest look at my academic record, including my cumulative GPA, science and math GPA, and nursing GPA?
2. If my GPA is not as competitive as I would like, have I developed a realistic plan to strengthen my academic profile before applying?
3. Am I viewing my GPA as a permanent limitation, or as one part of my application that I can continue to improve?
4. Have I demonstrated recent academic success that reflects the student I am today rather than the student I was years ago?
5. What specific courses could I take to strengthen my science and math GPA and demonstrate my readiness for graduate-level work?
6. If I apply this cycle and am not offered an interview, what academic steps could I take over the next year to become a more competitive applicant?
7. Beyond improving my GPA, what other areas of my application—such as ICU experience, certifications, leadership, or interview preparation—could I strengthen to present the strongest possible application?
8. Am I making decisions based on short-term convenience, or am I investing the time needed to become the strongest applicant and future nurse anesthetist I can be?

Why 3–5 Years of ICU Experience Matters Before Anesthesia School

One of the most common questions I hear is, *"How much ICU experience do I really need before applying?"* While many schools list a minimum requirement of one year, I have long encouraged applicants to view that as exactly what it is—a minimum, not necessarily the ideal.

Clinical expertise develops over time. There is simply no substitute for repeatedly caring for critically ill patients, managing emergencies, and learning from both successes and mistakes. Every vasoactive medication you titrate, every ventilator adjustment you make, every difficult family conversation you navigate, and every crisis you help manage adds another layer to your clinical judgment. Experience cannot be accelerated—it must be earned.

Over the years, I have become convinced that nurses with three to five years of high-quality ICU experience often enter anesthesia school with several important advantages. First, they tend to perform better academically because it may be months before they independently care for critically ill patients again while immersed in classroom learning. Their bedside experiences remain fresh and provide a framework for understanding the advanced physiology and pharmacology they are studying.

Second, the National Board of Certification and Recertification for Nurse Anesthetists (NBCRNA) has reported that candidates with more critical care experience are more likely to pass the National

Certification Examination (NCE) on their first attempt. This reinforces what many educators observe: a strong clinical foundation supports academic success.

Third, as our profession continues to distinguish itself through nursing expertise, the depth of ICU experience remains one of the defining characteristics of nurse anesthetists. Our nursing education and bedside experience shape the way we assess patients, recognize subtle changes, communicate with interdisciplinary teams, and make complex clinical decisions. Those experiences become part of your professional identity.

Finally, there is a level of professional maturity that simply cannot be taught in a classroom. Confidence without arrogance, humility, effective communication, leadership, and the ability to remain calm during a crisis are developed over years—not weeks or even months. You have to live half a century like me to REALLY appreciate what I am trying to get at. Even if you just want to dismiss my geriatric notion, I can guarantee you that those qualities that only come with time will serve you throughout anesthesia school and continue to define you as a CRNA long after graduation.

Why Is ICU Experience Preferred Over Emergency Department or Nurse Practitioner Experience?

One of the most common questions I receive is why nurse anesthesiology programs place such a strong emphasis on intensive care unit (ICU) experience instead of emergency department (ED) or nurse practitioner (NP) experience. The answer lies in the type of clinical thinking required in anesthesia. While emergency nurses are experts at rapid assessment, stabilization, and managing a broad spectrum of undifferentiated patients, anesthesia providers spend hours continuously managing a single critically ill patient whose physiology changes minute by minute. Similarly, nurse practitioners develop advanced skills in diagnosis, treatment planning, and longitudinal patient management, but many NP roles do not provide the continuous bedside management of mechanically ventilated, hemodynamically unstable patients that is central to anesthesia practice.

The ICU provides repeated exposure to advanced physiology and pharmacology that closely parallels the work of a CRNA. ICU nurses continuously titrate vasoactive medications, interpret invasive hemodynamic monitoring, manage mechanical ventilation, respond to rapidly changing patient conditions, and make minute-to-minute clinical decisions based on subtle physiologic changes. This constant immersion develops the pattern recognition, vigilance, and critical thinking that anesthesia providers rely on every day in the operating room.

This is not to suggest that emergency nurses or nurse practitioners are less skilled clinicians. They simply develop expertise in different areas of healthcare. Every specialty has its own knowledge base and strengths. Nurse anesthesiology programs are looking for applicants whose recent clinical experience most closely aligns with the responsibilities of providing an anesthetic. For that reason, high-acuity ICU experience remains the gold standard for preparing future nurse anesthesiology residents and ultimately safe, independent CRNAs

What about Neonatal and Pediatric ICU Experience?

Another question I am frequently asked is whether Pediatric Intensive Care Unit (PICU) or Neonatal Intensive Care Unit (NICU) experience is acceptable preparation for nurse anesthesiology school.

As a pediatric CRNA myself, I have tremendous respect for the knowledge and clinical judgment developed in both of these specialties. Some of the finest CRNAs I have ever worked with began their careers in the PICU or NICU. Caring for critically ill infants and children requires exceptional assessment skills, attention to detail, and the ability to recognize subtle changes in a patient's condition long before they become emergencies.

That said, not every nurse anesthesiology program views these experiences the same way.

Some programs readily accept PICU and NICU experience as qualifying critical care experience, while others prefer or require applicants to have experience caring for critically ill adults. Their reasoning is understandable. The majority of anesthesia care in most programs involves adult patients, and faculty may feel that adult ICU experience provides a stronger foundation for learning adult physiology, pharmacology, and disease processes.

Neither perspective is inherently right or wrong—it simply reflects differences in program philosophy and curriculum.

For that reason, if your experience is primarily in a PICU or NICU, do not assume every school will automatically consider you eligible. Review each program's admission requirements carefully, and if the information is unclear, contact the admissions office directly. Most programs are happy to clarify whether your experience meets their expectations before you spend time and money applying.

If your heart is in pediatric critical care, do not assume you have chosen the wrong path. Many outstanding CRNAs—and many outstanding pediatric CRNAs in particular—began exactly where you are. The key is finding a program whose admissions philosophy aligns with your experience and career goals.

Why is 3-5 years of ICU experience important?

1. Critical Thinking Isn't Learned Overnight

One of the greatest gifts the ICU gives you is the opportunity to develop clinical judgment. Early in your career, you often recognize when something is wrong because someone else tells you. After several years, you begin to recognize it yourself—sometimes before the monitor alarms, before the laboratory results return, or before a patient's condition obviously deteriorates. You learn to anticipate problems instead of simply reacting to them.

As a nurse anesthetist, every patient encounter requires constant assessment and decision-making. The ability to quickly identify subtle physiologic changes and intervene appropriately is one of the most important skills you will possess. That level of thinking is developed through repeated exposure to critically ill patients over time.

2. Complex Physiology Becomes Second Nature

During your first year in the ICU, much of your energy is spent learning how to survive each shift. By years three through five, you have likely cared for hundreds of mechanically ventilated patients, titrated countless vasoactive medications, managed invasive monitoring, interpreted arterial blood gases, and cared for patients with multi-organ failure.

Concepts such as:

- Mechanical ventilation
- Vasoactive infusions
- Hemodynamic monitoring

- Advanced pharmacology
- Continuous renal replacement therapy
- Shock physiology

become increasingly familiar through repetition.

When these concepts become second nature, you can devote your energy in anesthesia school to learning anesthesia rather than relearning critical care.

3. Technical Skills Become Automatic

Repetition builds confidence.

Experienced ICU nurses become highly proficient with procedures and technology, including IV placement, arterial lines, central venous catheters, medication titration, infusion pumps, invasive monitoring equipment, and troubleshooting complex devices.

When these technical skills become automatic, your mental energy can shift toward learning airway management, anesthesia equipment, regional anesthesia, and the many other new skills required during training.

4. Professional Maturity Cannot Be Taught in a Classroom

One of the biggest differences I notice between applicants with one year of ICU experience and those with several years is professional maturity.

After years of caring for critically ill patients, you learn how to communicate effectively with physicians, respiratory therapists, pharmacists, surgeons, consultants, patients, and families. You learn how to remain calm during emergencies, prioritize competing demands, advocate for your patients, and function as part of a high-performing team.

These are not skills developed by reading a textbook. They are developed by living them, one shift at a time.

Anesthesia school is demanding, both academically and emotionally. Professional maturity becomes one of the greatest predictors of resilience during those challenging months.

5. Pattern Recognition Creates Clinical Instinct

Experienced ICU nurses often describe having a "gut feeling" that something isn't right.

What appears to be intuition is actually pattern recognition developed over hundreds or even thousands of patient encounters.

You begin to recognize subtle trends before they become obvious:

- A slight change in mental status

- A gradual increase in vasopressor requirements
- Small ventilator changes
- Minor laboratory abnormalities
- Tiny shifts in vital signs

These seemingly insignificant findings often signal significant deterioration.

Anesthesia providers rely heavily on this same ability. Every anesthetic requires continuous observation and early recognition of changing physiology. Clinical instincts are not inherited—they are earned through experience.

6. Experience Makes the Transition Easier

Anesthesia education is unlike anything most nurses have previously experienced. The pace is rapid, expectations are high, and the amount of information can feel overwhelming.

Students who enter with several years of ICU experience generally have greater confidence in their clinical foundation. They are not necessarily "smarter," but they often have more mental bandwidth available because they already understand the language of critical illness.

Rather than trying to remember why norepinephrine works or how pressure-controlled ventilation differs from volume-controlled ventilation, they can focus on integrating anesthesia-specific concepts into knowledge they already possess.

Experience Matters More Than Time Alone

Although I encourage applicants to gain three to five years of ICU experience, I also recognize that not all experience is created equal.

One nurse may spend three years taking the sickest patients on the unit, volunteering for challenging assignments, serving on committees, precepting new nurses, earning certifications, and continually asking questions.

Another nurse may work the same number of years while remaining in a relatively comfortable routine with limited exposure to complex patients.

The calendar alone does not create expertise.

Ask yourself:

- Am I caring for the sickest patients available?
- Am I volunteering for difficult assignments?
- Do I understand *why* I am making clinical decisions?
- Am I seeking feedback from experienced colleagues?
- Am I continuing to grow every shift?

Those are the experiences that truly prepare you for anesthesia school.

Final Thoughts

As a Program Director, I have reviewed thousands of applications and watched hundreds of students progress through anesthesia school. While every student is unique, I have consistently observed that applicants with deeper ICU experience often transition more smoothly into the demands of anesthesia education. They arrive with stronger clinical judgment, greater confidence, and a professional maturity that serves them well throughout the program.

There is no prize for becoming a CRNA as quickly as possible.

The ICU is not simply a hurdle to clear before anesthesia school. It is where you develop the clinical judgment, confidence, technical ability, and professional identity that will define you for the rest of your career.

Every additional year spent intentionally growing as a critical care nurse is an investment—not only in your success as a student, but in the safety of the patients you will one day care for as an independent Certified Registered Nurse Anesthetist.

My final thought... One Year Makes You Eligible. Three to Five Years Often Makes You Ready.

Reflection Questions

1. Why do I want to become a CRNA, and am I allowing myself enough time to build the strongest possible clinical foundation before applying?

2. Looking back over the past year, how has my clinical judgment grown? Can I identify specific situations where I recognized a patient's deterioration earlier than I would have early in my ICU career?

3. Am I actively seeking out the sickest patients and the most challenging assignments, or have I become comfortable in my current routine?

4. Which critical care concepts still make me uncomfortable? What can I do over the next six months to strengthen those areas?

5. If I started anesthesia school tomorrow, what aspects of critical care would I feel confident about, and what areas would I struggle with?

6. How do I respond to stressful situations? Do I remain calm, communicate effectively, and prioritize patient safety under pressure?

7. Beyond technical skills, how have I grown professionally as a nurse? In what ways have I become a better communicator, teammate, mentor, or leader?

8. Am I viewing my ICU experience as a requirement to complete, or as an opportunity to become the best anesthesia provider I can be?

9. What experiences, certifications, committees, leadership opportunities, or educational activities could I pursue over the next year to continue developing as a critical care nurse?

10. Imagine yourself five years from now as a practicing CRNA. Looking back, what ICU experiences do you think you will be most grateful that you had before starting anesthesia school?

Letters of Recommendation

Letters of recommendation, or professional references, are a part of nearly every nurse anesthesiology program's application process. While the format varies from school to school, the goal is the same: to help admissions committees understand who you are as a professional from the perspective of those who have worked with you.

At Saint Mary's University of Minnesota, we ask applicants to have professional references complete Likert-scale evaluations rather than traditional narrative letters. We require one evaluation from a current supervisor and another from a healthcare professional who has firsthand knowledge of the applicant's clinical practice.

The evaluation focuses on professional behaviors such as whether the applicant:

- Interacts well with peers
- Is able to self-direct
- Acts professionally
- Solves problems logically
- Makes ethical decisions
- Accepts criticism well
- Takes responsibility for their actions

- Is organized
- Functions well during a crisis
- Is dependable

NursingCAS, which many nurse anesthesiology programs use, asks very similar questions. While individual schools may modify the format slightly, the themes are remarkably consistent. Programs are trying to determine whether you possess the professional characteristics necessary to succeed in an exceptionally demanding educational environment.

Choosing the Right References

One of the most common mistakes applicants make is assuming that anyone with an impressive title will write a strong recommendation. That is not necessarily true. A charge nurse or physician who genuinely knows your practice is often a far better choice than someone in a leadership position who has interacted with you only a handful of times.

Before listing someone as a reference, have an honest conversation with them. Rather than simply asking, "Will you write me a recommendation?" consider asking:

"Do you feel you know my practice well enough to provide me with a strong recommendation for nurse anesthesiology school?"

This wording gives the individual an opportunity to decline if they do not feel they can enthusiastically support your application. While that conversation can feel uncomfortable, it is far better to receive an honest answer than a mediocre evaluation that could weaken your application.

Talking With Your Manager

Many applicants dread asking their manager to serve as a reference. Some worry that their supervisor will be disappointed to lose a strong nurse or that discussing graduate school will create tension in the workplace.

In my experience, most managers are supportive when approached professionally. Remember that your manager is also invested in your long-term career development. Be respectful, communicate your goals clearly, and give them plenty of notice before application deadlines.

At the same time, be thoughtful about who you ask. If you have unresolved performance issues or a strained relationship with a supervisor, address those concerns before requesting a recommendation. Your references should be people who genuinely want to see you succeed, not individuals who may use the evaluation as an opportunity to express unrelated frustrations.

Program Directors Notice Patterns

One evaluation rarely determines an admissions decision. Instead, admissions committees look for patterns.

If every evaluator independently describes you as dependable, calm under pressure, organized, and eager to learn, that consistency strengthens your application considerably. Likewise, if multiple references identify concerns about professionalism, communication, accountability, or accepting feedback, those patterns carry significant weight.

We also notice patterns across organizations. As program directors, we become familiar with how managers and leaders from various hospitals complete evaluations over time. Some supervisors consistently rate everyone highly, while others are much more conservative in their scoring. After reviewing hundreds—or even thousands—of applications, those tendencies become apparent. We evaluate your recommendations within that broader context rather than relying solely on the raw scores.

Ultimately, strong recommendations are earned over months and years of consistently demonstrating professionalism, humility, teamwork, accountability, and clinical excellence. Long before you begin filling out applications, your reputation is already being built through every shift you work.

The Application Essay

Nearly every nurse anesthesiology program includes one or more application essays, and there is a good reason for that. While your GPA, résumé, certifications, and interview help us understand your accomplishments, your essays allow us to understand *you*. They demonstrate your ability to communicate effectively, organize your thoughts, reflect on your experiences, and express why you are pursuing one of the most challenging and rewarding professions in healthcare. Success in a doctoral nurse anesthesiology program requires strong written communication, and your application essays provide an early glimpse into that ability.

In recent years, the rapid growth of artificial intelligence (AI) has changed the admissions landscape. Every admissions committee is now faced with the challenge of determining whether an essay truly reflects the applicant's own thinking and writing. While AI can produce polished sentences, it often produces essays that are generic, impersonal, and remarkably similar from one applicant to the next. The essays that stand out are not necessarily the most eloquent—they are the ones that are authentic. We want to hear *your* voice, *your* experiences, and *your* reflections.

As a program director who receives over 400 applications, we need to quickly determine who took the time to actually write their essay. As part of this work, our program evaluates every essay submitted for A.I. use. This is the breakdown of the 2025 applications.

Overall AI Use Summary

- **Total applicants analyzed:** 271
- **Nearly half (51%)** of essays show **AI use above 60%,** suggesting substantial reliance on AI tools for writing or editing.
- **One in four applicants (25%)** appear to have written their essays largely without AI assistance.
- The **most common high-AI threshold values** were exactly **100%, 85%, and 77%**, which may indicate use of generative systems that produce detectable uniform outputs.
- **Several applicants with 0% AI use** still scored competitively on essay ratings, suggesting authenticity does not necessarily correlate with lower quality.

One of the most common misconceptions applicants have is that they need to write the "perfect" essay. Admissions committees are not looking for perfection. We are looking for insight, maturity, self-awareness, and evidence that you can think critically about your experiences. A sincere essay with genuine reflection is almost always more compelling than a flawlessly written essay that could have been generated by anyone—or anything.

Building a Strong Essay

What can you do to ensure your essay is as strong as possible? Start by asking people you trust to read it and provide honest, constructive feedback. Choose individuals who know you well enough to tell you whether your essay truly reflects who you are—not just whether it is grammatically correct. A trusted mentor, colleague, faculty member, or friend can often identify areas that need clarification or suggest examples that better highlight your strengths.

Expect to go through multiple drafts. Writing is a process, and your first draft is rarely your best. Each revision gives you an opportunity to refine your message, strengthen your examples, and ensure your responses directly answer the question being asked.

Perhaps most importantly, the writing process is an opportunity for self-reflection. As you revise, you will often gain a deeper understanding of your own motivations, strengths, and areas for growth. That self-awareness will not only make your essay stronger—it will also prepare you for the interview, where you'll be asked to expand on many of the same themes.

In the following pages, I have included examples of both weaker and stronger responses to common nurse anesthesiology application essay prompts. The weaker examples are not unrealistic; in fact, they resemble many essays submitted by well-intentioned applicants each year. The stronger examples illustrate the qualities that admissions committees value most: authenticity, reflection, specificity, and personal growth. As you read them, don't focus on copying the words. Instead, pay attention to the differences in storytelling, depth of reflection, and the way each essay answers the question being asked. Those are the qualities that will help your own voice stand out.

Example Essay Question #1: Why do you want to become a Certified Registered Nurse Anesthetist (CRNA)?

Discuss:

- What draws you specifically to nurse anesthesiology (not just advanced practice nursing)?
- What experiences have confirmed this decision?
- What do you understand about the realities and responsibilities of the profession?

Weak Essay Example

I have wanted to become a CRNA for a long time because I enjoy helping people and I want to continue advancing my nursing career. I have always enjoyed learning new things and challenging myself, and I believe becoming a CRNA is the next logical step for me. I have worked hard throughout my nursing career, and I think this profession will allow me to continue making a difference in patients' lives while also achieving my professional goals.

As an ICU nurse, I have cared for many critically ill patients. I enjoy taking care of patients who are very sick because every day is different and there is always something new to learn. I have become comfortable managing ventilators, vasoactive medications, and working with physicians and other members of the healthcare team. These experiences have helped prepare me for graduate education and have increased my confidence as a nurse.

I have also had the opportunity to shadow a CRNA. During that experience I observed several surgeries and was impressed by everything the CRNA was responsible for. I enjoyed watching the procedures and seeing how the CRNA interacted with patients before surgery. It was interesting to watch the induction of anesthesia and to see how the patient was carefully monitored throughout the procedure. The experience confirmed that this is what I want to do.

One of the reasons I am interested in becoming a CRNA is because I enjoy science. I have always liked physiology and pharmacology, and I believe nurse anesthesia combines these subjects in a way that is both interesting and rewarding. I know that anesthesia requires a great deal of responsibility, and I am willing to work hard to become successful.

I also appreciate the autonomy that CRNAs have. They are respected members of the healthcare team and are trusted to care for patients independently. I believe this level of responsibility would be both challenging and fulfilling. I enjoy making decisions and thinking critically, and I believe nurse anesthesia would allow me to continue developing those skills.

I understand that anesthesia school will be very difficult and require many hours of studying. I know there will be stressful situations and that I will need to remain calm under pressure. I have always been a hard worker and I am confident that I can succeed if I am given the opportunity.

Overall, I believe becoming a CRNA is the right career choice for me. It combines my interest in science, patient care, and professional growth. I look forward to continuing my education and eventually providing safe anesthesia care to patients while making a positive impact on their lives.

Why this essay is weak

This is the kind of essay that admissions committees read dozens of times every cycle.

It isn't *bad*—it's simply **forgettable**.

It tells us:

- "I like science."

- "I like helping people."
- "I shadowed a CRNA."
- "I like autonomy."

Unfortunately, almost every applicant says those same things. The essay contains almost no personal reflection, no memorable story, no evidence that the applicant truly understands the profession, and very little insight into *why this person* wants to become a CRNA.

Strong Essay Example

The first time I truly understood what a CRNA did, it wasn't during a dramatic airway or a complicated trauma. It was during a five-minute conversation with a frightened patient before surgery.

As an ICU nurse, I had grown comfortable managing critically ill patients. I understood vasopressors, ventilators, and invasive monitoring. I enjoyed solving physiologic problems and working in an environment where every decision mattered. But while shadowing a CRNA, I watched something different happen. Before touching an IV or administering medication, the CRNA sat beside an anxious patient, listened to her concerns, explained the anesthetic plan in language she understood, and transformed fear into trust. Moments later, that same provider seamlessly transitioned into managing a complex anesthetic, constantly anticipating physiologic changes before they became problems.

That experience changed my understanding of nurse anesthesiology.

I realized that anesthesia is much more than administering medications or placing an endotracheal tube. It is the unique responsibility of guiding patients safely through one of the most vulnerable moments of their lives. Every decision has immediate consequences, and every patient deserves someone who is completely prepared, attentive, and accountable.

Working in the ICU has reinforced that calling every day.

One of my most memorable patients was a middle-aged man who rapidly deteriorated from septic shock. Over several hours I titrated multiple vasoactive infusions, adjusted ventilator settings in collaboration with the intensivist, monitored laboratory trends, and continually reassessed his response to treatment. Although the interventions themselves were important, what stayed with me was how quickly his condition changed and how essential it was to anticipate problems before they occurred. I learned that waiting until something becomes a crisis is often too late.

That lesson closely mirrors what attracts me to anesthesia. The best anesthesia providers are not simply reacting to changes—they are constantly thinking several steps ahead. They understand physiology so thoroughly that they recognize subtle warning signs before instability develops. That level of vigilance is what I aspire to.

I also understand that becoming a CRNA means accepting tremendous responsibility. Patients place complete trust in the anesthesia provider at a moment when they are unable to advocate for themselves. That responsibility cannot be taken lightly. It demands lifelong learning, humility, emotional resilience, and the confidence to make difficult decisions while remaining open to continual growth.

I am under no illusion that anesthesia school will be easy. I expect it to be one of the most academically and emotionally demanding experiences of my life. I also recognize that graduation is not the finish line. Medicine evolves continuously, and exceptional CRNAs remain students throughout their careers. That commitment to lifelong learning is something that excites me rather than intimidates me.

Ultimately, I am pursuing nurse anesthesiology because it brings together everything I value most about healthcare. It requires deep scientific knowledge, calm decision-making under pressure, compassionate patient care, and unwavering accountability. More importantly, it provides the opportunity to care for patients during some of the most critical moments of their lives. That is both an incredible privilege and a profound responsibility—one that I hope to earn through dedication, humility, and hard work.

Why this essay works

This essay succeeds because it answers the question beneath the question. The admissions committee wants to evaluate the candidate's professional calling and motivation behind their decision to go to anesthesia school.

Instead of simply saying, *"I like science and autonomy,"* it demonstrates:

- **Specific experiences** rather than general statements.
- **Reflection** instead of a chronological resume.
- An understanding of **what CRNAs actually do** beyond technical skills.
- Knowledge of the **responsibility, vigilance, and lifelong learning** required in the profession.
- A clear, authentic voice that feels personal rather than generic.

Most importantly, when an admissions committee finishes reading this essay, they remember the applicant. That is ultimately the goal of every application essay.

Example Essay Question #2: What is a personal limitation or growth area you are actively working on?

Describe:

- How it has impacted you
- What steps you are taking to improve
- Why this awareness matters in your future anesthesiology practice

Weak Essay Example

One of my biggest limitations is that I am a perfectionist. Throughout my nursing career I have always held myself to a very high standard. I want everything to be done correctly, and I often spend extra time making sure that my work is accurate. While I believe this has helped me become a good nurse, it has also caused me unnecessary stress because I worry about making mistakes.

Being a perfectionist has affected me in several ways. Sometimes I spend too much time reviewing my work or double-checking tasks that I have already completed. I also place a lot of pressure on myself to perform well, which can make me anxious. I have learned that healthcare is unpredictable and that not everything goes according to plan. Despite this, I still find myself wanting everything to be perfect.

I have been working on improving this by reminding myself that no one is perfect. I have learned to trust my education and my experience. I also ask questions whenever I am unsure about something, and I seek feedback from my coworkers and supervisors. Their encouragement has helped me become more confident in my abilities.

As an ICU nurse, I have become more comfortable making decisions under pressure. I understand that there are times when quick action is more important than achieving perfection. Although I still like to do things correctly, I recognize that patient care requires flexibility and teamwork.

I know anesthesia school will be challenging, and I expect there will be times when I will need to accept constructive criticism. I believe my willingness to learn will help me continue growing throughout the program. I also understand that becoming a CRNA requires lifelong learning, and I am excited for the opportunity to continue developing my skills.

Overall, I continue to work on balancing my desire for perfection with the realities of healthcare. I believe this growth will help me become a better student and ultimately a better CRNA.

Why this essay is weak

This is probably the single most common "weakness" admissions committees read.

The problem is not that perfectionism can't be a weakness—it certainly can be. The problem is that the applicant never demonstrates **true vulnerability**.

The essay:

- never tells a story.
- never shows consequences.
- never demonstrates meaningful personal growth.
- feels like a safe answer designed to impress rather than an honest reflection.

When every applicant claims to be a perfectionist, the essay becomes forgettable.

Strong Essay Example

One of the greatest areas of growth in my professional life has been learning that competence does not mean having all the answers—it means knowing when to ask for help.

Early in my ICU career, I believed that asking too many questions would make me appear inexperienced. I wanted to prove that I belonged in a high-acuity environment, so I often tried to solve problems independently before seeking assistance. While this approach came from a desire to be capable, I eventually realized that it could also delay learning and, more importantly, limit opportunities to benefit from the experience of others.

One shift early in my career fundamentally changed my perspective. I was caring for a patient whose vasopressor requirements were increasing despite aggressive treatment. I spent considerable time reviewing laboratory values, adjusting medications within my scope, and trying to determine why the patient was deteriorating. Eventually, I asked a more experienced nurse to review the situation with me. Within minutes, she identified subtle clinical changes that suggested worsening right ventricular failure rather than simply progressing septic shock. Her observations changed our discussions with the intensivist and ultimately altered the patient's management.

Driving home after that shift, I realized my hesitation to seek another perspective had nothing to do with confidence—it had everything to do with pride.

Since then, I have intentionally worked to replace the mindset of needing to appear knowledgeable with a commitment to continual learning. I actively seek feedback after difficult cases, ask experienced colleagues how they would approach complex situations, and participate in debriefings even when they are optional. I have found that the nurses and physicians I respect most are not the ones who pretend to know everything. They are the ones who are curious enough to recognize that medicine is too complex for any individual to master alone.

This change has also affected how I mentor newer nurses. I make a point of creating an environment where questions are welcomed rather than judged. I remember how intimidating it felt to admit uncertainty, and I want others to know that asking thoughtful questions is a sign of professionalism, not weakness.

I believe this lesson is particularly important in nurse anesthesiology. Anesthesia providers make independent decisions with significant consequences, but true autonomy does not mean practicing in isolation. Safe anesthesia care requires humility, continual reassessment, and the confidence to consult colleagues whenever a situation exceeds one's experience. In fact, I believe one of the most dangerous providers is the one who believes they no longer have anything to learn.

This growth has also changed how I view graduate education. I am not applying because I think I have mastered critical care nursing. I am applying because I recognize how much more there is to learn. I want to be challenged by faculty, learn from experienced CRNAs, and continually refine my clinical judgment. I expect to make mistakes during my education—not mistakes that compromise patient safety, but mistakes that become opportunities for reflection and improvement under careful supervision.

Today, I still strive for excellence, but I no longer equate excellence with having every answer. Instead, I define it as maintaining intellectual humility, seeking feedback without defensiveness, and remaining committed to lifelong growth. I believe that mindset will not only help me succeed in a doctoral nurse anesthesiology program, but will ultimately make me a safer, more thoughtful anesthesia provider.

Why this essay works

This essay feels authentic because the applicant admits a genuine limitation without undermining their ability to become a CRNA. It also shows that the applicant understood what the admissions committee was looking for: **Self-Awareness and Growth.** It also demonstrates several qualities admissions committees value:

- The weakness is believable and professionally relevant.
- The applicant tells a specific story rather than making broad statements.
- The essay shows measurable growth and a change in behavior.
- It connects the lesson directly to the practice of nurse anesthesiology.

- Most importantly, it demonstrates humility—a trait that is essential for safe anesthesia practice and one that faculty consistently value in successful students and future CRNAs.

Reflection Questions:

1. What story do you want your admissions essay to tell about you that is not already evident from your GPA, resume, or transcripts?
2. Who are three people you trust to provide honest, constructive feedback on your essay? Why did you choose them?
3. After reading your essay, would someone who knows you well say, "Yes, this sounds exactly like you"? Why or why not?
4. Have you clearly answered every part of the essay prompt, or have you drifted into telling the story you wanted to tell instead?
5. What strengths, experiences, or personal qualities are demonstrated through your examples rather than simply stated?
6. If an admissions committee member only remembered one thing about your essay six months later, what would you want that to be?

7. What did you learn about yourself during the writing process that you did not fully appreciate before you began?
8. After completing your final draft, read it aloud. Where does it sound natural and authentic, and where does it sound forced or unlike your own voice?

CHALLENGE REFLECTION QUESTION:

If your essay were the only piece of your application an admissions committee could read, would it convince them that you belong in nurse anesthesiology? If not, what is still missing?

The Interview: Looking for Reasons to Say Yes

Many applicants approach the interview believing they have to convince the admissions committee that they are capable of succeeding in nurse anesthesiology school. In reality, most candidates who make it to the interview have already demonstrated the academic ability and clinical foundation needed to be successful. I truly believe that the vast majority of ICU nurses who apply could complete a nurse anesthesiology program and become excellent CRNAs. The purpose of the interview is not to identify the 95% who can succeed—it is to identify the small percentage of applicants who, for one reason or another, may not yet be ready for the unique demands of the profession. We are looking for concerns related to professionalism, judgment, integrity, communication, self-awareness, or interpersonal skills that may not be apparent on paper. In other words, we are looking for reasons to protect both the profession and our future patients. If you come to the interview prepared, authentic, humble, and able to thoughtfully discuss your experiences, you have already overcome one of the biggest hurdles in the admissions process.

Practice With Purpose

Like any important performance, a successful interview requires practice—but there is a difference between being well prepared and sounding rehearsed. Admissions committees want to get to know the real you, not listen to memorized answers. Practice enough that you become comfortable discussing your experiences naturally, but avoid trying to script every response.

One of the best ways to prepare is to record yourself answering common interview questions. Watching the recording can help you identify distracting habits, improve your eye contact, eliminate filler words, and evaluate whether your answers sound authentic. Ask trusted friends, colleagues, mentors, or CRNAs to conduct mock interviews and challenge you with follow-up questions. You can also search online for common medical school, graduate healthcare, or CRNA interview questions to broaden your preparation.

Throughout your ICU career, keep a notebook of meaningful patient experiences, leadership opportunities, ethical dilemmas, communication challenges, and clinical situations that taught you important lessons. Reviewing these examples before an interview will make it much easier to recall stories that demonstrate your growth and critical thinking.

On interview day, bring several professional copies of your resume to offer each interviewer, even if they already have one in your application file. It reflects professionalism and allows them to easily reference your accomplishments during the conversation.

Finally, prepare thoughtful questions for the interviewers. Take time to review the program's website beforehand so you do not ask questions that are already answered there. Instead, ask about the program's culture, student support, clinical experiences, mentorship, faculty philosophy, or what characteristics distinguish the students who are most successful. Thoughtful questions demonstrate genuine curiosity and show that you have done your homework before arriving.

Sample Questions

1. What initially sparked your interest in becoming a nurse anesthetist, and what experiences have confirmed that this is the right career path for you?

Strong Answer

"I first became interested in nurse anesthesiology after working with CRNAs during my ICU orientation. What initially caught my attention was the level of autonomy and the depth of physiology involved, but I knew I didn't want to pursue the profession based on observation alone. Over the past three years, I've shadowed CRNAs multiple times, spoken with several providers about both the rewards and challenges of the profession, and intentionally sought out the sickest patients in my ICU. I've learned that nurse anesthesiology isn't just about intubation or medications—it's about taking complete responsibility for a patient during one of the

most vulnerable moments of their life. That responsibility is exactly what attracts me."

Weak Answer

"I've always wanted to do more with my nursing career. CRNAs seem to have a great job, they're respected, and I've heard they have a good work-life balance. I think I'd really enjoy it."

---

2. Walk me through your nursing career so far.

Strong Answer

"I graduated from nursing school in 2021 and began working in a mixed medical-surgical ICU. During my first year I focused on becoming comfortable managing ventilators, vasopressors, CRRT, and caring for septic shock patients. As I became more confident, I volunteered to precept new nurses, joined our unit practice council, earned my CCRN, and became ultrasound IV certified. Those experiences have helped me become more confident clinically while also improving my leadership and communication skills."

Weak Answer

"I've worked in the ICU for about two years. I take care of ICU patients, give medications, and work with the physicians. I've learned a lot and think I'm ready for anesthesia school."

3. Describe a particularly challenging patient or clinical situation.

Strong Answer

"I cared for a patient with rapidly worsening septic shock who required multiple vasopressors, mechanical ventilation, and continuous dialysis. During the shift, the patient's blood pressure deteriorated despite escalating therapy. I recognized subtle changes early, notified the intensivist, prepared medications before they were requested, and helped coordinate care with respiratory therapy and pharmacy. Although the patient ultimately did not survive, I learned the importance of anticipating problems, communicating early, and remaining calm during rapidly evolving situations."

Weak Answer

"I've had lots of difficult patients. Usually we just work together as a team and get through it. It taught me that teamwork is important."

---

4. What steps have you taken to prepare yourself professionally and personally for anesthesia school?

Strong Answer

"I've tried to prepare in several ways. Professionally, I earned my CCRN, completed graduate chemistry, shadowed multiple CRNAs, and have continued to seek high-acuity assignments. Personally, I've reduced my debt, discussed the financial commitment with my family, built a support system, and adjusted my work schedule so I can focus fully on school. I understand this will require significant sacrifices, and I've tried to prepare for those before classes even begin."

Weak Answer

"I know school will be hard, but I'm motivated. It's hard to say what it will be like, so, I'll figure things out once I get in."

---

5. Describe your communication style.

Strong Answer

"I try to communicate directly, respectfully, and calmly. When someone is upset, my first goal is to understand why they're frustrated before trying to solve the problem. I don't assume they're upset with me personally. I ask questions, listen first, and then focus on finding a solution that keeps the patient at the center of the discussion."

Weak Answer

"I'm pretty easy-going. I don't really find myself involved in conflicts at work."

---

6. Tell me about a healthcare systems problem you recognized. How did you address it?

Strong Answer

"Our unit experienced repeated delays in obtaining emergency blood products. Rather than simply accepting it, several coworkers and I gathered examples, discussed the issue with leadership, and participated in developing a revised process with the blood bank. While the changes weren't perfect, turnaround times improved. That experience taught me that bedside nurses can improve systems when they approach problems constructively."

Weak Answer

"Our hospital has lots of problems. Management doesn't really listen, so there's not much you can do. I just try to watch out for myself as much as possible."

---

7. Tell me about a time you received difficult feedback.

Strong Answer

"Early in my ICU career, my preceptor told me I tended to focus so much on completing tasks that I sometimes missed the bigger clinical picture. At first that was difficult to hear because I was working hard. After reflecting on it, I realized she was right. I began reviewing each patient's diagnosis before every shift, anticipating complications, and asking more 'why' questions during rounds. Looking back, that feedback helped accelerate my clinical growth."

Weak Answer

"I honestly can't think of any major negative feedback. I've always gotten good evaluations."

---

8. How do you manage stress?

Strong Answer

"I've learned that stress management has to be intentional. I prioritize sleep, regular exercise, and spending time with my family. During particularly stressful periods, I rely on organization, meal preparation, and maintaining routines instead of sacrificing healthy habits. I also recognize when I need support and am comfortable asking for help before I become overwhelmed."

Weak Answer

"I usually just deal with stress when it happens. Once school starts, I'll probably just study as much as possible."

---

9. What questions do you have for me?

Strong Answer

"I'd love to hear what qualities consistently distinguish your strongest students from those who struggle. How does your program support students academically and personally? Finally, what advice would you give someone who wants to excel rather than simply graduate?"

Weak Answer

"How much vacation do students get? Where do your students go for clinical?

I think these examples accomplish something important. The weak answers aren't "bad" because they're incorrect—they're bad because they lack depth, insight, and self-reflection. That's exactly what admissions committees notice. Conversely, the strong answers don't rely on extraordinary accomplishments; they demonstrate maturity, preparation, thoughtful reflection, and a genuine understanding of the profession. Those are the qualities that consistently make applicants memorable.

Beware of Overconfidence

Confidence is an important quality in healthcare. Patients need providers who can make decisions under pressure, communicate clearly, and remain calm in difficult situations. Overconfidence, however, is something entirely different—and it can be one of the quickest ways to derail an interview.

One of the biggest misconceptions applicants have is believing they need to convince the admissions committee that they already think like a CRNA. You do not. You are applying to become a student, not an expert. We expect you to have knowledge gaps. In fact, we would much rather interview someone who is humble, curious, and eager to learn than someone who believes they already have all the answers.

Overconfidence often appears in subtle ways. Applicants may exaggerate their role in patient care, speak dismissively about coworkers or physicians, insist there was only one correct way to manage a clinical situation, or answer every question with complete certainty despite limited experience. These behaviors raise concerns because they suggest a lack of self-awareness. In nurse anesthesiology, confidence without humility can be dangerous.

The strongest applicants project quiet confidence. They openly acknowledge what they know, admit what they do not know, and demonstrate a genuine desire to continue learning. They recognize that becoming a CRNA is a journey of lifelong professional growth, not a destination they have already reached.

Remember, admissions committees are not looking for perfection. They are looking for applicants who are teachable. Humility, professionalism, and intellectual curiosity are far more impressive than trying to prove you already know everything.

Follow Up With a Thank-You

Your interview doesn't end when you walk out the door. Sending a thoughtful thank-you email within 24 to 48 hours is a simple but professional way to express your appreciation for the interviewer's time and reinforce your interest in the program. Keep your message brief and sincere. Thank the interviewers for the opportunity, mention one or two aspects of the conversation that were particularly meaningful to you, and reaffirm your enthusiasm for joining their program. Avoid trying to introduce new accomplishments or persuade the committee to change its opinion of your application. The purpose of a thank-you note is simply to demonstrate professionalism, gratitude, and respect. While a thank-you email alone will not earn you admission, failing to acknowledge the time and effort your interviewers invested can be a missed opportunity to leave a positive final impression.

Reflection Questions

1. Why do admissions committees place so much emphasis on the interview, even after reviewing your academic record and application?

2. Think about your own motivation for becoming a CRNA. Could you explain it in a way that is personal, specific, and memorable?

3. What three ICU patient experiences best demonstrate your critical thinking, communication skills, and professional growth?

4. How have you prepared academically, professionally, financially, and personally for the demands of nurse anesthesiology school?

5. Describe a time you received difficult feedback. How did it change the way you practice today?

6. What qualities distinguish confidence from overconfidence during an interview? How can you demonstrate humility while still presenting yourself as a strong candidate?

7. If someone asked you to describe your communication style, what examples would you use to support your answer?

8. What questions would you ask a nurse anesthesiology program that could not be answered by reading its website?

9. If you recorded yourself answering interview questions today, what aspects of your communication would you expect to improve?

10. Is your resume polished, professional, and ready to hand to every interviewer? If not, what changes should you make before interview season?

11. Have you started keeping a notebook of meaningful ICU experiences? What stories would you include today that demonstrate leadership, resilience, teamwork, or clinical judgment?

12. Imagine the interview ended today. What three things would you want the admissions committee to remember most about you?

Part IV: Preparation for School

Financing Your Nurse Anesthesiology Education

For many aspiring nurse anesthesiologists, financing graduate school is one of the greatest challenges in the application process. Tuition, fees, and the inability to work full-time during an intensive doctoral program often require students to rely on federal and private educational loans. In recent years, the graduate student loan landscape has changed significantly, with ongoing legislative proposals and policy changes affecting borrowing limits, repayment options, and loan forgiveness programs. Because these programs continue to evolve, it is essential that applicants seek the most current information directly from their university's financial aid office and the U.S. Department of Education before making financial decisions.

While the cost of nurse anesthesiology education is substantial, graduates have historically enjoyed strong employment opportunities and earning potential, making the investment worthwhile for many students. Fortunately, nurse anesthesiology graduates have historically demonstrated excellent repayment outcomes because they enter a profession with strong demand and competitive salaries. The greatest financial risk is often not the loan itself—it is borrowing money and then being unable to complete the program. This is one more reason to take your academic preparation seriously and fully commit yourself to your studies from the very beginning. Understanding your financing options early will help you develop a realistic financial plan and reduce unnecessary stress throughout your educational journey.

The number one rule you must follow is: *Do not start living like a CRNA before you are one.*

Can You Work During Nurse Anesthesiology School?

One of the most common questions applicants ask is whether they can continue working while enrolled in nurse anesthesiology school. The honest answer is yes—you are legally allowed to work. In fact, programs generally cannot prohibit you from maintaining employment. However, that does not mean working is advisable.

Nurse anesthesiology education is one of the most academically and clinically demanding professional programs in healthcare. You will spend long days in the classroom, laboratory, simulation center, and operating room, followed by evenings and weekends studying, preparing for cases, completing assignments, and recovering from the mental and physical demands of training. There simply are not many hours left in the week.

Every year, I meet applicants who confidently tell me they plan to continue working one or two shifts each pay period. Occasionally, a student is able to make that work for a period of time. More often, however, those shifts become the first thing to disappear when examinations become more challenging, clinical responsibilities increase, or fatigue begins to affect learning.

The students who struggle the most are often those who underestimate the workload and overestimate the amount of free time they will have. Unfortunately, I have seen more than one student realize too late that they did not devote enough time early in the program to build a strong foundation. Nurse anesthesiology education is cumulative—each concept builds upon the last. When students fall behind in the beginning, catching up can become increasingly difficult, and in some cases, they ultimately face academic dismissal. It rarely happens overnight. Instead, it often develops gradually until the gap between what they know and what they need to know becomes too large to overcome. Schools are not responsible for making sure you study each day—that responsibility belongs to you.

Think of nurse anesthesiology school as a full-time job—and then some. Your primary responsibility is to become a safe, competent anesthesia provider. If working begins to interfere with your academic performance, clinical preparation, or personal well-being, it is no longer serving your long-term goals. Before you commit to outside employment, have an honest conversation with your support system, develop a realistic financial plan, and remember that your education is an investment in a career that will last decades.

How Much Time Should You Expect to Spend Studying?

One of the biggest adjustments students make when they begin nurse anesthesiology school is learning how to manage their time. A good rule of thumb used throughout higher education is that for every one credit hour you take, you should expect approximately one hour of direct interaction with the program each week. This includes lectures, laboratory experiences, simulations, seminars, and other scheduled learning activities. In addition, you should plan to spend two to three hours studying outside of class for every credit hour.

Let's put that into perspective. If you are enrolled in a 14-credit semester, you can expect approximately 14 hours each week interacting directly with the program. You should then plan on spending at least another 28 to 42 hours studying, reviewing material, preparing for class, and completing assignments. That means you are already committing 42 to 56 hours each week to your education before you factor in commuting, meals, exercise, family responsibilities, household chores, appointments, or simply getting enough sleep.

For many critical care nurses, this is a dramatic shift. In the ICU, you are accustomed to working long shifts where you are constantly moving, solving problems, and caring for patients. Success in graduate school requires a different type of endurance. You must learn to spend long periods sitting, reading, reviewing concepts, and thinking deeply about complex material. That transition can be surprisingly difficult at first. Time management becomes one of the most important skills you will develop, and students who establish effective study habits early are often the ones who thrive throughout the program.

Reflection Questions:

1. Have you developed a realistic financial plan for completing nurse anesthesiology school? If not, what steps do you need to take before applying?
2. If you plan to work during school, what specific factors will you use to determine whether your job is helping or hindering your academic success?
3. What expenses in your current lifestyle could you reduce or eliminate before beginning your program?
4. Who will be part of your support system during graduate school, and have you discussed the financial and personal sacrifices that will be required?
5. Using the "one hour in class and two to three hours studying per credit" guideline, estimate how many hours each week you will devote to school during a 14-credit semester. What activities in your current schedule would need to change?

6. How do you currently study? Which of your study habits are likely to help you succeed in graduate school, and which habits will need to change?

7. What distractions are most likely to interfere with your study time, and what strategies can you put in place to minimize them?

8. Have you ever experienced falling behind academically because you underestimated the workload? What did you learn from that experience?

9. What does "treating school like a full-time job" mean to you, and how will you demonstrate that mindset from your first day in the program?

10. Looking back five years from now, what sacrifices do you think will have been worth making to achieve your goal of becoming a CRNA?

Know Yourself Before You Know Anesthesia

Preparing for nurse anesthesiology school is about far more than improving your GPA, earning certifications, or building a competitive resume. Those things certainly matter, but they are only part of the journey. The transition from critical care nurse to nurse anesthesiology student—and ultimately to anesthesia provider—requires intentional personal growth. The students who thrive are often those who have spent time understanding themselves: how they think, how they respond to stress, how they communicate, where their greatest strengths lie, and perhaps most importantly, where they still have room to grow.

Unlike many personality assessments that focus primarily on behaviors, the Enneagram attempts to uncover the motivations that drive those behaviors. Although its exact origins are debated, the Enneagram is an ancient system of personality that has been studied and refined for decades in psychology, leadership, education, and personal development. Rather than simply describing what people do, it seeks to explain why they do it. Two nurses may respond to the same clinical situation in exactly the same way, yet for completely different reasons. One may be motivated by a desire to do everything perfectly, another by a need to protect others, and another by a desire to be recognized as highly competent. The outward actions may look identical, but the internal motivations are different. Understanding those motivations is where real personal growth begins. As you move through this assessment, try to look beyond what you do and instead ask yourself why you do it. That level of self-awareness can be incredibly valuable as you prepare for the challenges of nurse anesthesiology education and the lifelong practice of anesthesia.

One of the greatest gifts you can give yourself before starting school is honest self-awareness. Every personality brings unique strengths to the profession, and every personality also carries blind spots that become more apparent under the intense pressures of anesthesia education. This section is not intended to place you into a box or suggest that one personality type is better than another. Rather, it is designed to help you begin the important work of self-reflection. As you complete the Enneagram assessment, review the common personality traits, and consider the suggested growth areas, challenge yourself to ask not, "Which type am I?" but "How can I become the healthiest version of myself?"

Nurse anesthesiology school has a remarkable way of exposing both our strengths and our weaknesses. The more work you do on yourself before you arrive, the more resilient, adaptable, and emotionally intelligent you will become—not only as a student, but as a future CRNA. Your greatest competition is not the other applicants. It is becoming a better version of yourself than you were yesterday.

Enneagram Quiz for Critical Care Nurses

Instructions:

Rate each statement on a scale from 1 (Not at all true) to 5 (Very true) based on how you typically feel and act in your critical care nursing role.

Category 1

___ I insist on precision and proper technique in high-risk procedures.

___I get frustrated when policies or best practices are not followed.

___I hold myself to high moral and professional standards, even under stress.

___I feel responsible for maintaining high levels of care even when others don't

___I notice errors or inefficiencies in protocols and I feel compelled to correct them.

___I struggle when colleagues don't follow procedures carefully.

___I take pride in doing things the right way and maintaining high standards.

___I want to create structure and integrity in the world around me.

___I want to improve the world and make it more ethical and fair.

___I become rigid and insist on “the right way” to do things

Category 2

___I regularly put my patients' emotional and physical needs ahead of my own.

___ I notice when team members are struggling and try to support them quietly.

___ I feel most fulfilled when I know I’ve made someone feel cared for.

___ I go out of my way to support patients and colleagues even if it adds to my workload

___ I often anticipate the needs of others before they express them.

___ It’s hard for me to say no when someone asks for help, even if I am exhausted.

___ I’m deeply empathetic and lead by creating emotional connection

___ I need to be helpful and supportive so others feel safe around me

___I become overly accommodating and may neglect my own needs.

Category 3

___I'm driven to excel and be seen as competent, even in emergencies.

___I like being known as a high-performer or go-to nurse in the unit.

___I often track my own metrics or benchmarks to gauge performance.

___I take pride in being recognized for my performance or leadership.

___I strive to be seen as competent, efficient, and reliable in my team.

___I often compare my productivity to others in the workplace.

___I inspire others with my achievements and confidence.

___I want to be admired for my leadership and success.

___I overwork and try to prove my worth through success.

Category 4

___I feel emotionally affected by my patients' stories long after a shift ends.

___I often find deeper meaning or personal growth through intense situations.

___I need time to process emotions after critical incidents.

___I'm deeply affected by the emotional weight of patient care.

___I value authenticity and emotional connection in my work relationships

___I sometimes feel differently from my coworkers, like I experience things more deeply.

___I desire to be unique and deeply understood.

___I get emotional or moody if I feel misunderstood.

___At work I value being real over fitting in with the group

Category 5

___I prefer having detailed clinical knowledge to feel confident in care.

___I sometimes emotionally detach to stay focused in life-or-death moments.

___I spend free time researching conditions, procedures, or equipment.

___I value evidence-based practice and prefer to make decisions based on data.

___I enjoy learning about new treatments, techniques, or technologies in healthcare

___I sometimes withdraw emotionally to conserve energy during long or difficult shifts.

___I prefer figuring out complex problems on my own

___I am curious, innovative, and always thinking about what is next.

___I withdraw and overthink before making a move

Category 6

___I am constantly scanning for what could go wrong and preparing for it.

___I trust systems, protocols, and experienced team members in crises.

___I often double-check everything to ensure patient safety.

___I often worry about what could go wrong and try to prepare for every scenario

___I am very loyal to my team and expect the same in return

___I rely heavily on rules and guidelines to make decisions

___I'm a loyal and responsible leader, but I often anticipate what could go wrong.

___I strive for certainty and security in every decision I make.

___I worry about being betrayed or unsupported.

Category 7

___I stay upbeat during high-pressure situations to keep morale up.

___I enjoy fast-paced environments where every day is different.

___I tend to avoid burnout by staying busy or shifting focus.

___I try to keep the mood light, even in stressful situations

___I get excited about trying new specialties, shifts, or roles in healthcare

___I sometimes take on too much because I enjoy staying busy and involved.

___I'm energetic, optimistic, and enjoy keeping things upbeat and moving forward.

___I strive to create freedom and excitement in the world around me.

___I avoid discomfort by distracting myself or others with new ideas.

Category 8

___I advocate strongly for my patients, especially when they can't.

___I push back against decisions I believe aren't in the best interest of care.

___I take charge in critical situations without waiting for permission.

___I stand up for patients and colleagues if I think they're being treated unfairly.

___I dislike being micromanaged and prefer to take the lead when possible.

___I'm not afraid to challenge authority if I believe it's in the wrong

___When I am in charge, I lead with a clear vision and expect others to follow.

___I feel most alive when I'm in control and protecting others.

___I take charge and might become too forceful or blunt.

Category 9

___I try to maintain harmony among staff during stressful shifts.

___I'm good at staying calm and grounded even during codes.

___I often go along with others to avoid workplace tension.

___I try to avoid conflict in the workplace whenever possible.

___I'm often the one others come to for calm, steady support.

___I tend to go along with group decisions, even if I have a different opinion.

___I try to keep the peace and lead by ensuring harmony among the team

___I want to avoid conflict and make sure everyone feels included.

___I become overly accommodating and may neglect my own needs.

Put the total points for each category (type) here:

Enneagram Type	Total Score
Type/ Category 1 – The Reformer	____________
Type/ Category 2 – The Helper	____________
Type/ Category 3 – The Achiever	____________
Type/ Category 4 – The Individualist	____________
Type/ Category 5 – The Investigator	____________

Type/ Category 6 – The Loyalist __________

Type/ Category 7 – The Enthusiast __________

Type/ Category 8 – The Challenger __________

Type/ Category 9 – The Peacemaker __________

Results Interpretation

• Your highest-scoring type is your likely Enneagram personality at work.

• The second-highest may be a wing or strong secondary influence.

• All types have strengths in critical care—this just highlights how you approach stress, care, and team dynamics.

Enneagram Personality Traits for Critical Care Nurses

Type 1 – The Reformer (The Ethical Perfectionist)

• Detail-oriented and precise during high-risk procedures.

• Driven by ethical standards and clinical excellence.

• Insists on adherence to best practices and protocols.

• Feels responsible for ensuring high-quality care at all times.

• Corrects inefficiencies and errors to protect patient outcomes.

• Leads with integrity and moral clarity.

• Struggles with internal pressure to be perfect.

• Values structure, accountability, and transparency.

• Can be perceived as overly critical or rigid under stress.

• Calm under pressure when clear protocols are in place.

Type 2 – The Helper (The Compassionate Caregiver)

• Highly empathetic and emotionally attuned to patient needs.

• Goes above and beyond to care for patients and team members.

• Anticipates the needs of others before they are spoken.

• Finds fulfillment in making others feel safe and supported.

• Often neglects their own needs while caring for others.

• Builds trust through emotional connection and presence.

• Creates a warm, comforting environment in high-stress settings.

• Struggles to say no, even when overwhelmed.

• Supports colleagues quietly and reliably.

• Seeks harmony through caregiving and connection.

Type 3 – The Achiever (The Performer)

• Driven to perform well and exceed expectations.

• Strives for recognition as a competent and efficient nurse.

• Motivated by success, achievement, and professional growth.

• Often serves as a role model or high performer on the unit.

• Measures success through outcomes, benchmarks, or metrics.

• May overwork to prove worth and reliability.

• Excels in fast-paced, competitive environments.

• Values confidence, capability, and upward mobility.

• Can be image-conscious or avoid vulnerability.

• Inspires others through ambition and leadership presence.

Type 4 – The Individualist (The Deep Feeler)

• Deeply affected by patients' stories and emotional suffering.

• Seeks authenticity and emotional connection with patients.

• Values meaningful, one-on-one interactions in care.

• Feels uniquely sensitive to the emotional atmosphere of the unit.

• Finds purpose and self-understanding through intense experiences.

• Needs time to process after emotionally charged situations.

• May feel misunderstood or emotionally isolated at work.

• Creative and insightful in navigating patient-centered care.

• Leads with emotional depth and sincerity.

• Can become withdrawn or moody when emotionally overwhelmed.

Type 5 – The Investigator (The Specialist)

• Prefers in-depth clinical knowledge and evidence-based practice.

• Emotionally detaches in crisis to maintain clinical focus.

• Researches new treatments, technologies, and data.

• Solves problems independently and methodically.

• Enjoys mastering new skills and acquiring expertise.

• Withdraws to recharge during overwhelming shifts.

• Values competence and intellectual clarity in care.

• Can be perceived as aloof or emotionally distant.

• Thinks strategically and avoids unnecessary drama.

• Leads through insight, precision, and innovation.

Type 6 – The Loyalist (The Defender)

• Scans for risks and prepares thoroughly for worst-case scenarios.

• Values systems, protocols, and experienced leadership.

• Loyal and dependable under pressure.

• Double-checks details to ensure patient safety.

• Feels secure when clear guidelines are in place.

• Worries about what could go wrong and plans accordingly.

• Protects their team and expects loyalty in return.

• Can become anxious or overly cautious in ambiguity.

• Trusts authority but questions when necessary.

• Leads by ensuring safety, preparedness, and follow-through.

Type 7 – The Enthusiast (The Energizer)

• Brings high energy and optimism to high-stress situations.

• Thrives in dynamic, fast-paced environments.

• Stays upbeat and keeps morale high during long shifts.

• Enjoys trying new roles, specialties, or challenges.

• Avoids burnout by shifting focus or staying busy.

• Can take on too much to avoid discomfort or boredom.

• Creative and spontaneous under pressure.

• Encourages flexibility and adaptability in care teams.

• Can struggle with follow-through on less exciting tasks.

• Leads with enthusiasm, resilience, and resourcefulness.

Type 8 – The Challenger (The Protector)

• Takes charge quickly and decisively in crises.

• Advocates fiercely for patients and staff fairness.

• Pushes back against unsafe or unethical decisions.

• Values autonomy and resists micromanagement.

• Unapologetically direct and assertive.

• Feels most alive when protecting others.

• Can be perceived as intimidating or overly forceful.

• Leads with strength, vision, and confidence.

• Challenges authority when care is at stake.

• Ensures others feel protected and empowered.

Type 9 – The Peacemaker (The Stabilizer)

• Stays calm and grounded in emergencies.

• Works to maintain harmony among team members.

• Often acts as a mediator during conflict.

• Avoids confrontation unless absolutely necessary.

• Reliable, steady, and comforting presence on the unit.

• Tends to defer to others to preserve group cohesion.

• Neglects own needs to keep the peace.

• Values inclusiveness and team well-being.

• Can become disengaged under extreme stress.

• Leads by fostering unity, trust, and calm.

Enneagram Growth Areas for Critical Care Nurses

Type 1 – The Reformer (The Ethical Perfectionist)

• Letting go of perfection and accepting that “good enough” is sometimes okay

• Delegating tasks and trusting others' approaches

• Managing internal criticism and self-judgment

• Being flexible in rapidly changing situations

• Allowing room for mistakes without shame

Type 2 – The Helper (The Compassionate Caregiver)

• Setting boundaries and saying no without guilt

• Recognizing and addressing personal needs

• Avoiding burnout from over-helping or people-pleasing

• Accepting appreciation without needing constant affirmation

• Letting others struggle or solve problems independently

Type 3 – The Achiever (The Performer)

• Slowing down and focusing on genuine connection over performance

• Being vulnerable and authentic instead of always projecting competence

• Avoiding burnout from overwork or chasing recognition

• Accepting failure or imperfection as part of learning

• Letting go of comparison with others

Type 4 – The Individualist (The Deep Feeler)

• Regulating emotional intensity during high-stakes care

• Avoiding isolation or over-identification with suffering

• Focusing on tasks even when emotionally overwhelmed

• Letting go of the need to feel unique or misunderstood

• Finding meaning in teamwork, not just personal experience

Type 5 – The Investigator (The Specialist)

• Engaging emotionally with patients and colleagues

• Sharing knowledge and asking for help when needed

• Avoiding over-analysis or emotional detachment

• Managing energy proactively during long or demanding shifts

• Practicing presence instead of retreating into research or planning

Type 6 – The Loyalist (The Defender)

• Trusting intuition and not over-relying on external authority

• Managing anxiety and fear-based thinking

• Letting go of worst-case scenario fixation

• Being open to change or uncertainty in protocols

• Developing confidence in decision-making under pressure

Type 7 – The Enthusiast (The Energizer)

• Slowing down to process difficult emotions and trauma

• Following through on less exciting but essential tasks

• Facing discomfort instead of avoiding it with distraction

• Respecting structure and limitations

• Avoiding overcommitment and being present with suffering

Type 8 – The Challenger (The Protector)

• Practicing gentleness and vulnerability

• Listening deeply before asserting control

• Trusting team members and encouraging shared leadership

• Recognizing how forcefulness can impact others emotionally

• Balancing strength with empathy

Type 9 – The Peacemaker (The Stabilizer)

• Speaking up with their own perspective

- Taking initiative instead of deferring to others
- Staying engaged during conflict instead of avoiding it
- Prioritizing personal needs and goals
- Making decisions instead of going with the flow

Reflection Questions

1. What did you learn about yourself from the Enneagram assessment that surprised you? How might this insight help you become a stronger graduate student and future CRNA?
2. The Enneagram focuses on motivations rather than behaviors. Why is understanding *why* you respond a certain way more valuable than simply recognizing *what* you do?
3. What are your greatest strengths as identified by your Enneagram type? How will these qualities benefit you in nurse anesthesiology school and clinical practice?
4. What growth areas are associated with your personality type? Which one do you believe could have the greatest impact on your success if left unaddressed?
5. Think about a recent stressful situation in the ICU. How did your personality influence the way you communicated, made decisions, or interacted with your team?

6. Who in your life knows you well enough to provide honest feedback? What are one or two questions you could ask them to better understand your blind spots?

7. Self-awareness is a lifelong process, not a one-time assessment. What habits or practices (such as journaling, seeking mentorship, mindfulness, coaching, or regular self-reflection) could help you continue growing throughout graduate school?

8. How do you typically respond to constructive criticism? Does your reaction help or hinder your growth? What strategies can you use to become more receptive to feedback?

9. Imagine yourself on the first day of anesthesia school. What aspects of your personality do you hope remain your greatest strengths, and what aspects do you hope you have intentionally developed before you arrive?

10. If your family, coworkers, or closest friends were asked to describe your communication style under stress, what do you think they would say? Would their description match how you see yourself?

Professional Communication and Email Etiquette

Professional communication begins long before you step into the operating room. In fact, I would argue that it starts as soon as you begin communicating with a program as you plan your educational journey. Every email, phone call, classroom interaction, and clinical conversation contributes to your professional reputation.

As a graduate student, you are no longer communicating as an undergraduate learner—you are communicating as a future healthcare provider. People notice your professionalism long before they evaluate your clinical skills.

One expectation I have of every student is that faculty members are addressed professionally in all forms of communication. Whether you are sending an email, speaking after class, or leaving a voicemail, use appropriate titles unless you have been specifically invited to do otherwise. A simple "Dr. Smith," "Professor Jones," or "Mr./Ms." demonstrates respect and professionalism. Likewise, emails to faculty should never read like text messages. Avoid abbreviations, slang, emojis, one-line messages, or overly casual language. Take a few moments to write complete sentences, proofread your message, and ensure your communication reflects the professional you are becoming.

Email etiquette is another skill that will serve you well throughout your career. Before sending an email, ask yourself whether it truly requires an immediate response. Unless your message involves an urgent issue affecting patient care or an immediate academic concern, try to avoid sending emails during evenings, weekends, or holidays. Faculty members value personal time just as you do. Most email programs now allow you to use a "Schedule Send" feature, which lets you write your message when it is convenient for you while having it delivered during normal business hours. It is a small gesture that demonstrates respect for the recipient's time.

Before clicking "Send," take one final look at your email. Is your subject line clear? Have you included all of the information the recipient needs to answer your question? Did you proofread for spelling and grammar? Have you addressed the correct person? Finally, pay close attention to who should be copied on the message. There are times when it is appropriate—and expected—to carbon copy (CC) faculty, clinical coordinators, administrative staff, or supervisors so that everyone involved has the same information. Thoughtful use of the CC line promotes transparency, prevents miscommunication, and ensures the appropriate people remain informed. At the same time, avoid unnecessarily copying large groups of people who do not need to be included.

Strong communication is a hallmark of exceptional clinicians. Patients, surgeons, anesthesiologists, nurses, and faculty all rely on providers who communicate with clarity, respect, and professionalism. Developing these habits now will not only make you a stronger graduate student, but will also help establish the professional reputation that follows you throughout your career.

Reflection Questions:

1. Think about a recent professional interaction. Did your communication reflect the professionalism you want to be known for as a future CRNA? If not, what would you do differently next time?
2. How do you typically respond when you are overwhelmed or under stress? Do you communicate your needs early, or do you tend to withdraw, become frustrated, or try to handle everything on your own? How might this affect your success in graduate school?
3. What is one communication habit you would like to improve before starting nurse anesthesiology school? Develop a specific plan for how you will practice and strengthen that skill over the next six months.

Preparing Your Family and Friends for the Journey

One of the biggest predictors of success in nurse anesthesiology school has very little to do with academics. It has everything to do with the people surrounding you.

I often tell prospective students that nurse anesthesiology school is a jealous mistress. It will demand your time, your energy, your attention, and at times even your emotional capacity. For the next three years, there will be periods when school simply has to come first. That does not mean your family is less important—it means you are making a temporary investment that will provide lifelong rewards for everyone involved.

Before classes ever begin, sit down with the people who matter most in your life. Talk honestly about what the next three years will look like. Explain that there will be long days, weekends spent studying, early mornings, clinical call, examinations, and times when you may not be as available as you have been in the past. Help them understand that your absence is not a reflection of your love or commitment to them. It is a reflection of the commitment required to become a safe anesthesia provider.

Support systems do not happen by accident—they are built intentionally. Discuss practical responsibilities before school starts. Who will prepare meals? Who will pick up the children from school or daycare? Who will care for pets? How will household chores be divided? What will happen if you are studying for a major examination while your spouse is traveling for work? These conversations may not be exciting, but they prevent unnecessary stress when life inevitably becomes busy.

It is equally important to establish expectations with your friends. There will be birthdays, weddings, vacations, sporting events, and social gatherings that you simply cannot attend. Some friends will understand immediately. Others may not. Remember that saying "no" for a season is not selfish—it is necessary. The people who truly care about you will still be there when graduation arrives.

At the same time, do not allow school to consume every aspect of your identity. Schedule time for the people who matter most. A dinner with your family, a walk with your spouse, attending your child's school event, or a cup of coffee with a close friend can recharge you far more effectively than another hour of distracted studying. Success in graduate school is not about studying every waking moment; it is about using your time intentionally.

Finally, don't forget to thank the people who are making sacrifices alongside you. While you are earning the degree, your family and closest friends are also carrying part of the burden. They may take on additional responsibilities, miss vacations, or simply accept that your schedule revolves around exams and clinical rotations. Never let those sacrifices go unnoticed. A handwritten note, a heartfelt conversation, or a simple "thank you" can go a long way toward strengthening the relationships that sustain you throughout this journey.

Remember, you are not attending nurse anesthesiology school alone. Although only one person receives the diploma, an entire support system helps make that achievement possible. Invest in those relationships before school begins, nurture them throughout the program, and celebrate together when you finally cross the stage as a Certified Registered Nurse Anesthetist.

The Family Meeting Checklist

Before nurse anesthesiology school begins, schedule a dedicated conversation with your spouse, partner, family members, or anyone who will be part of your support system. Use the questions below to guide your discussion.

While this is set up to be a moment in time (while you are reading this book), this document should be considered to be a framework that you return to at least annually.

Time Expectations

☐ Does everyone understand the time commitment required for nurse anesthesiology school?

☐ Have we discussed that evenings, weekends, and holidays may often include studying?

☐ Are we prepared for long clinical days, early mornings, and occasional call responsibilities?

Financial Planning

☐ Have we created a realistic budget?

☐ Do we understand how our income may change during school?

☐ Have we discussed educational loans and our financial expectations?

☐ what are our costs that we know we need to consider (child care, house payment, car payment, etc.)

Household Responsibilities

☐ Who will prepare meals?

☐ Who will handle grocery shopping?

☐ Who will manage laundry and house cleaning?

☐ Who will take care of yard work, home maintenance, or snow removal?

☐ Have we discussed hiring help if needed?

Children and Family Responsibilities

☐ Who will handle school drop-offs and pick-ups?

☐ Who will attend children's activities when I cannot?

☐ Who is our backup for childcare if an emergency arises?

☐ Have we explained this journey to our children in an age-appropriate way?

Study Environment

☐ Do I have a quiet place dedicated to studying?

☐ Have we agreed on uninterrupted study times?

☐ Does everyone understand when I should not be interrupted unless it is truly important?

Communication

☐ How can my family best encourage me during stressful periods?

☐ How will we let each other know when we are feeling overwhelmed?

☐ Have we agreed to discuss concerns early instead of letting frustration build?

Relationships

☐ How will we intentionally protect time together?

☐ Can we schedule regular date nights, family dinners, or other meaningful activities?

☐ Have we accepted that missing some social events is a temporary sacrifice?

Your Support Team

☐ Who are the people I can call when I need encouragement?

☐ Who can help with childcare or household responsibilities if needed?

☐ Who will hold me accountable when I become discouraged?

Personal Wellness

☐ What will I do to protect my physical and mental health?

☐ How will I prioritize sleep, exercise, healthy eating, and stress management?

☐ What signs will tell me I need to ask for help?

Graduation Vision

Finally, ask everyone this question:

"Three years from now, when we walk across the graduation stage together, what do we hope we will say about how we supported one another through this journey?"

Keep your answers somewhere visible. Return to them throughout school, especially during difficult semesters. Your plan will evolve, but having these conversations before classes begin can prevent unnecessary conflict and strengthen the relationships that will carry you through one of the most challenging—and rewarding—experiences of your life.

Reflection Questions

1. Who are the three people who will have the greatest influence on your success during nurse anesthesiology school? Have you had an honest conversation with them about the time commitment and sacrifices that lie ahead?
2. What responsibilities outside of school (family, finances, household duties, childcare, work, etc.) are most likely to compete with your academic success? What plans can you put in place now to reduce those stressors?
3. How will you communicate with your family and friends when school becomes overwhelming? What expectations should you establish before classes begin?

4. Think about your current support system. What strengths does it already have, and where might you need additional help or resources?
5. What activities or relationships are most important to maintaining your physical and emotional well-being? How can you intentionally protect those throughout graduate school?
6. Imagine yourself six months into the program. What challenges do you think your family or partner will be experiencing, and what can you do now to prepare for them?
7. If your spouse, partner, family member, or closest friend were reading this chapter, what do you think they would say they need from you in order to successfully navigate this journey together?

Conclusion

Final Thoughts: The Journey Begins Now

If you have made it to the end of this book, congratulations. You have already taken an important step toward becoming the kind of applicant—and ultimately the kind of nurse anesthesiologist—our profession needs.

Throughout these chapters, I have tried to be honest with you. Admission to nurse anesthesiology school is competitive, and the journey is demanding. There will be moments of self-doubt, disappointment, exhaustion, and sacrifice. There will also be incredible moments of growth, confidence, achievement, and purpose. Every challenge you overcome will prepare you for the responsibility of one day caring for patients during some of the most vulnerable moments of their lives.

Remember that admissions committees are not searching for perfection. They are searching for potential. They want applicants who are academically prepared, clinically capable, emotionally mature, humble enough to continue learning, and resilient enough to persevere when things become difficult. Your experiences—both your successes and your failures—have shaped who you are. Learn from them, own them, and let them become part of your story.

As you move forward, continue to invest in yourself. Strengthen your clinical knowledge. Seek feedback. Ask thoughtful questions. Develop your leadership skills. Care for your physical and mental well-being. Nurture the relationships that will support you through graduate school. Most importantly, begin thinking and acting like the anesthesia provider you aspire to become. Professional identity does not begin on the first day of school—it begins the day you decide to pursue this profession.

Never lose sight of why you started. On the difficult days, remember the patient who inspired you, the mentor who believed in you, or the family member who encouraged you to take this leap. Purpose has a remarkable way of carrying us through seasons when motivation alone is not enough.

One day, perhaps sooner than you realize, you will walk into an operating room as a Certified Registered Nurse Anesthetist. You will earn the trust of patients, surgeons, nurses, and colleagues through your preparation, your vigilance, your compassion, and your professionalism. The work is challenging, but it is also one of the greatest privileges in healthcare.

I sincerely hope our paths cross someday as colleagues. Whether I meet you as an applicant, a student, a graduate, or a fellow CRNA, I look forward to welcoming you into this remarkable profession.

Until then, keep learning. Stay humble. Be curious. Support others. Lead with integrity. And never stop striving to become the provider your future patients deserve.

I believe in this profession. I believe in the future of nurse anesthesiology. And I believe there is a place for you in it.

I wish you the very best on your journey.

APPENDIX A: CALCULATING YOUR MATH AND SCIENCE GPA

This worksheet is used by the Nurse Anesthesiology Admissions Committee to calculate your science and math GPA, which is a component of the candidate selection process.

Please complete the worksheet using:

- Science and mathematics courses from the **most recent 90 credits of post-secondary coursework** and/or courses completed within the **last 10 years.** Please use the list on page 2 as your guide.
- **All nursing courses,** regardless of when they were taken

Additional guidelines:

- The Admissions Committee will **verify all calculations** and may adjust course inclusion after reviewing official transcripts
- **Do not include** pass/fail coursework
- **Do not include** separate laboratory courses in your GPA calculation

To calculate your science & math GPA, use the following steps:

1. List each completed course and the number of credits earned. Please list the required chemistry course for admission first.
2. Do not include courses currently in progress. List earned grades only.
3. If a course was repeated, list only the highest grade earned and do not include earlier attempts.
4. Multiply the number of credits by the grade to get the "Grade Points" for each course.
5. Add the Grade Points for each course together to get Total Grade Points.
6. Divide the Total Grade Value Points by the total number of Credits attempted

Grade	Grade Value	Grade	Grade Value
A	4.0	C	2.0
A-	3.67	C-	1.67
B+	3.33	D+	1.33
B	3.00	D	1.00
B-	2.67	D-	0.67
C+	2.33	F	0.00
Incomplete or audited courses should not be included			

Example - This is an example of how Saint Mary's University of Minnesota will calculate your GPA. Please note that the program has a list of courses that they will consider to be science & math (See Page 2).

Course	Credits	Earned Grade	Grade Value	Grade Value Points
Chem 101	4	A	4.0	16
Chem 102	1	A	4.0	4
Bio chem 103	3	A-	3.67	11.01
Nurs 201	4	B+	3.33	13.32
Nurs 202	3	A	4.0	12
TOTAL	15 credits			56.33 Total grade Value points

56.33 Total Grade Value points ÷ 15 credits Taken = 3.76 GPA in the math and sciences

The following categories represent **examples of courses that may be considered science or math.** Certain courses are intentionally left off this list.

The Nurse Anesthesiology admissions committee will make the final determination

Biology

- Anatomy
- Biology
- Biophysics
- Biotechnology
- Cell biology
- Ecology
- Entomology
- Genetics
- Histology
- Immunology
- Microbiology
- Molecular biology
- Neuroscience
- Pathophysiology
- Physiology

Chemistry

- Biochemistry
- Chemistry
- Organic Chemistry
- Physical chemistry
- Thermodynamics

Health Sciences

- Allied health
- Chiropractic
- Clinical Courses
- Dentistry
- Hearing and speech studies
- Kinesiology
- Nutrition
- Occupational therapy
- Optometry
- Osteopathy
- Physical therapy
- Physician assistant
- Public health
- Pharmacology & pharmacy
- Sports medicine
- Veterinary medicine

Mathematics

- All courses that have 'math' or 'mathematics' in the title
- Biostatistics
- Statistics

Nursing

- All courses that have 'nursing' in the title or as the course code (i.e., NUR, NURS, NRSG, etc.)
- Clinical courses (Theory and Experiences)
- Lifespan courses (maternal health, pediatrics, gerontology, population health, etc.)
- Ethics in Nursing
- Psychology and mental health for nurses (NOT general psychology)
- Statistics for Nurses

Physics

- General physics
- Medical physics
- Applied physics
- Mechanics
- Electricity and magnetism

Course Number	Course Name	School Name	Semester & Year Taken	Credits	Earned Letter Grade	Grade Value Points	Total Grade Value Points (grade value points x credits)
			Totals				

Total Credit Hours: ______
Total Grade Points: ______

Calculated Science & Math GPA: ______

Appendix B: Review Questions

Part I: Starting the Journey

"Who are you becoming?"

1. Why do you truly want to become a nurse anesthesiologist? If the salary disappeared tomorrow, would this still be the career you would choose? Why or why not?
2. What personal strengths do you already possess that will help you succeed in nurse anesthesiology school? Which areas will require intentional growth?
3. Think about the nurses and healthcare professionals you admire most. What qualities do they possess that you hope to emulate throughout your career?
4. What sacrifices will pursuing this goal require of you, and are you prepared to make them?

Part II: The School Search

"Finding the right fit."

1. Beyond location or reputation, what characteristics are most important to you in a nurse anesthesiology program?
2. How does your preferred learning style influence the type of educational environment in which you are most likely to succeed?
3. Which aspects of a program would you be willing to compromise on, and which are non-negotiable?

4. If you were interviewing a program instead of them interviewing you, what questions would you ask to determine whether it is the right fit?
5. When you imagine graduation day three years from now, what kind of clinician do you hope that program has helped you become?

Part III: The Application Process

"Presenting your best self."

1. If an admissions committee spent only one minute reviewing your application today, what impression would they likely form about you?
2. Which parts of your application best demonstrate your aptitude? Which best demonstrate your attitude?
3. What experiences have shaped your character more than your résumé can fully capture? How might you communicate those experiences authentically?
4. If you were denied admission this cycle, what constructive steps would you take to become a stronger applicant rather than becoming discouraged?
5. What does professionalism mean to you, and how can you demonstrate it consistently throughout the admissions process?

Part IV: Preparation for School

"Preparing for success—not just admission."

1. What aspects of your current life will need to change in order for you to be fully successful in graduate school?
2. Who will make up your support system during the next three years, and have you had honest conversations with them about the challenges ahead?
3. What habits do you need to build—or break—before classes begin?
4. How will you protect your physical health, mental well-being, and relationships while balancing the demands of anesthesia school?
5. At the end of your education, what do you hope patients, classmates, faculty, and colleagues will say about the kind of provider you became?

Final Reflection

Take a few minutes to write a letter to your future self. Imagine you are reading it on the day you graduate from nurse anesthesiology school.

- Why did you begin this journey?
- What obstacles do you expect to face?
- What values do you refuse to compromise?
- What kind of provider do you hope to become?
- What would you want your future self to remember on the hardest day of school?

Seal it away. Read it again on graduation day. You may discover that while your knowledge has changed dramatically, the person you hoped to become was already beginning to take shape long before your first day of class.

Educational Disclaimer

The information presented in this book is intended for educational and informational purposes only. Although every effort has been made to ensure the accuracy and currency of the information at the time of publication, healthcare, educational, and admissions practices evolve over time. Readers are encouraged to verify current standards, policies, and requirements directly with the appropriate organizations and individual nurse anesthesiology programs.

Nothing in this publication should be interpreted as legal, medical, financial, or other professional advice. The opinions expressed are those of the author and are based on professional experience and available evidence at the time of writing.

Limitation of Liability

The author and publisher disclaim any liability for any loss, injury, claim, or damage, whether direct, indirect, incidental, consequential, or otherwise, arising from the use of, or reliance upon, the information contained in this publication. Readers assume full responsibility for how they apply the material presented.

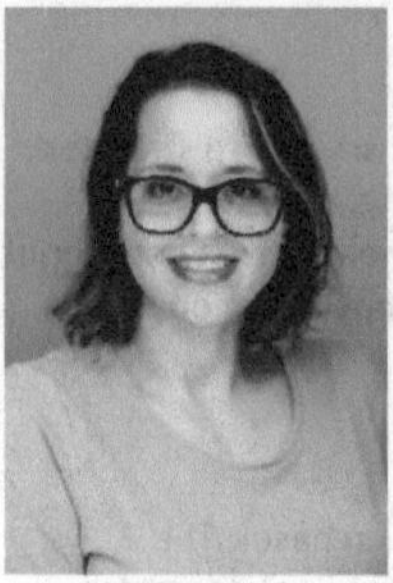

About the Author

Leah M. Gordon, DNP, APRN, CRNA is a nurse anesthetist, educator, and academic leader with more than two decades of experience in nursing and nurse anesthesiology. She serves as the Program Director of the Doctor of Nursing Practice in Nurse Anesthesiology program at Saint Mary's University of Minnesota, where she has helped develop one of the nation's leading doctoral programs and has mentored hundreds of aspiring CRNAs through the admissions process and beyond.

In addition to her academic leadership, Leah maintains an active clinical practice as a Certified Registered Nurse Anesthetist (CRNA), providing anesthesia care in outpatient settings. Remaining in clinical practice allows her to bring current, real-world experience into the classroom and ensures her teaching remains grounded in the realities of modern anesthesia care.

A passionate educator and national speaker, Leah has presented extensively on anesthesia practice, leadership, provider development, and professional resilience. She has served in numerous leadership positions within the Minnesota Association of Nurse Anesthetists as well as the Minnesota APRN Coalition, and has been recognized for her contributions to the profession, including the Brother Louis DeThomasis Award for Entrepreneurship and Integrity from Saint Mary's University of Minnesota and the Outstanding Professional Accomplishment Award from the Minnesota Association of Nurse Anesthetists.

Although she leads a graduate nurse anesthesiology program, Leah's journey was anything but traditional. With an undergraduate GPA that would have discouraged many aspiring applicants, she understands firsthand that successful providers are not defined by a single number, but by perseverance, growth, humility, and a commitment to excellence. That experience has shaped her holistic philosophy of admissions and her dedication to helping future providers recognize and develop their full potential.

The *Provider Mindset* series was created to give applicants honest, practical guidance from someone who has reviewed applications, conducted interviews, mentored students, and celebrated their success. Leah's goal is simple: to help future advanced practice providers become not only competitive applicants, but exceptional professionals.

Leah lives in Minnesota with her husband, Beau, their son, Grady, and their two-rescue Boston Terriers. When she isn't caring for patients or mentoring future providers, she enjoys writing, speaking, and advocating for the nurse anesthesiology profession.

www.ingramcontent.com/pod-product-compliance
Lightning Source LLC
LaVergne TN
LVHW040518210926
848480LV00007BA/1506
9798234139559